Veterinary Anesthesia

D0872872

The Practical Veterinarian

Veterinary Neurology
Shawn P. Messonnier, ISBN 0-7506-7203-X

Veterinary Anesthesia
Janyce L. Cornick-Seahorn, ISBN 0-7506-7227-7

Coming Soon

Veterinary Parasitology
Lora Rickard Ballweber, ISBN 0-7506-7261-7

Veterinary Toxicology
Joseph Roder, ISBN 0-7506-7240-4

Veterinary Dermatology
Karen A. Moriello, ISBN 0-7506-7299-4

Veterinary Oncology
Kevin A. Hahn, ISBN 0-7506-7296-X

Small Animal Dentistry
Paul Q. Mitchell, ISBN 0-7506-7321-4

Veterinary Anesthesia

Janyce L. Cornick-Seahorn, D.V.M., M.S., D.A.C.V.A., D.A.C.V.I.M.

Former Associate Professor of Anesthesiology, Department of Veterinary Clinical Sciences, Louisiana State University College of Veterinary Medicine, Baton Rouge; Medical Director, Vet-Scans.com Imaging Center, Lexington, Kentucky; Consultant, Veterinary Anesthesia Practice and Consultation, Georgetown, Kentucky

Series Editor
Shawn P. Messonnier, D.V.M.
Paws & Claws Animal Hospital, Plano, Texas

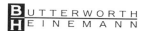

Boston   Oxford   Auckland
Johannesburg   Melbourne   New Delhi

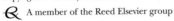
Every effort has been made to ensure that the drug dosage schedules within this text are accurate and conform to standards accepted at time of publication. However, as treatment recommendations vary in the light of continuing research and clinical experience, the reader is advised to verify drug dosage schedules herein with information found on product information sheets. This is especially true in cases of new or infrequently used drugs.

 Recognizing the importance of preserving what has been written, Butterworth–Heinemann prints its books on acid-free paper whenever possible.

 Butterworth–Heinemann supports the efforts of American Forests and the Global ReLeaf program in its campaign for the betterment of trees, forests, and our environment.

Library of Congress Cataloging-in-Publication Data
Cornick-Seahorn, Janyce L.
    Veterinary anesthesia / Janyce L. Cornick-Seahorn.
        p. cm. — (The Practical veterinarian)
    Includes bibliographical references (p.   ).
    ISBN 0-7506-7227-7 (alk. paper)
        1. Veterinary anesthesia. I. Title. II. Series.
    SF914 .C67 2000
    636.089'796—dc21   00-044452

British Library Cataloguing-in-Publication Data
A catalogue record for this book is available from the British Library.

The publisher offers special discounts on bulk orders of this book. For information, please contact:

Manager of Special Sales
Butterworth–Heinemann
225 Wildwood Avenue
Woburn, MA 01801-2041
Tel: 781-904-2500
Fax: 781-904-2620

For information on all Butterworth–Heinemann publications available, contact our World Wide Web home page at: http://www.bh.com

10 9 8 7 6 5 4 3 2 1

Printed in the United States of America

Contents

Series Preface

The Practical Veterinarian series was developed to help veterinary students, veterinarians, and veterinary technicians find answers to common questions quickly. Unlike larger textbooks, which are filled with detailed information and meant to serve as reference books, all the books in The Practical Veterinarian series are designed to cut to the heart of the subject matter. Not meant to replace the reference texts, the guides in our series complement the larger books by serving as an introduction to each topic for those learning the subject matter for the first time or as a quick review for those who already have mastered the basics of each subject.

The titles for the books in our series are selected to provide information for the most common subjects one would encounter in veterinary school and veterinary practice. The authors are experienced and established clinicians who can present the subject matter in an easy-to-understand format. This helps both the first-time student of the subject and the seasoned practitioner assess information often difficult to comprehend.

It is our hope that the books in The Practical Veterinarian series will meet the needs of readers and serve as a constant source of practical and important information. We welcome comments and suggestions that will help us improve future editions of the books in this series.

Shawn P. Messonnier, D.V.M.

Preface

Veterinary Anesthesia summarizes what I hope is practical, useful information for learning the basic and clinical principles and the daily practice of anesthesia. I would like to thank my husband, Tom, and my children, Brad and Sam, without whom this project would not have had such meaning. I would like to thank my parents, without whom I would not have had the opportunity to achieve my goals nor the desire to share my knowledge, as I hope I have in this endeavor.

I thank my mentor in anesthesia, Dr. Sandee Harts-field, who continues to be a friend and unending source of knowledge and common sense regarding the art of anesthesia. I thank my mentor in large animal internal medicine, Dr. Kent Carter, who instilled in me a logical and thorough approach to case management.

I also thank my editor, Leslie Kramer, whose optimism and enthusiasm gave me support every step of the way.

And, most of all, I thank God for my profession and the opportunity to accrue the information and knowledge that I feel are most pertinent to teach veterinary students and guide practitioners, many of whom I have been fortunate to interact with at some level of their careers.

The book is not comprehensive but includes those drug dosages, techniques, and procedures I feel are pertinent to the daily practice of veterinary medicine. Many of the recommendations and dosages are based on clinical experience, which I hope will complement and enhance the clinical practice of anesthesia.

J.L. C-S.

1

Introduction to Anesthesia and Patient Preparation

Anesthesia is defined as total loss of sensation in a body part or the whole body, induced by a drug or drug combination that depresses activity of nervous tissue peripherally (local and regional anesthesia) or centrally (general anesthesia). Anesthesia and chemical restraint are reversible processes essential to the practice of veterinary medicine, providing safe and effective patient immobilization to minimize stress and pain and facilitate a wide variety of procedures.

General Principles of Anesthetic Management

Regardless of species and procedure, these guidelines should be applied to all patients:

1. Critical evaluation of history, physical examination, and laboratory data. Know your patient!

2. Weigh the benefits of the procedure against the potential detrimental effects of anesthesia.

3. Stabilize and correct any identified abnormalities, if possible, prior to anesthesia.

4. Be organized to minimize anesthesia time.

5. Identify and prepare for potential complications.

6. Select the anesthetic protocol based on the patient and existing abnormalities.

7. Establish intravenous access whenever possible and feasible.

8. Secure and maintain a patent airway whenever possible and feasible.

9. Use supplemental oxygen when indicated, based on patient and duration of procedure.

10. Use a maintenance regimen that will minimize adverse effects.

11. Provide ventilatory support.

12. Monitor vital body systems, including cardiovascular, respiratory, and central nervous systems.

13. Identify and correct any abnormalities that arise during the anesthetic period.

14. Continue monitoring and support until vital signs are stable.

15. Use appropriate analgesia and sedation postoperatively to minimize pain and distress.

Patient Preparation

"For every mistake that is made for not knowing,
a hundred are made for not looking."

—Anonymous

Patient preparation includes evaluation of the signalment, history, and pertinent laboratory data that might affect the patient's response to anesthesia. Patients then can be categorized according to physical status, which helps in the selection of an anesthetic protocol and determines the likelihood (risk) for occurrence of a cardiopulmonary emergency during the anesthetic period (Table 1–1).

Physical examination should always include assessment of temperature, heart rate, respiratory rate, mucous membrane color and moistness, pulse quality, thoracic auscultation, and abdominal palpation, even in seemingly healthy patients. Normal values for a variety of species are listed in Table 1–2. Minimal laboratory data in physical status I patients should include packed cell volume (PCV) and total protein for all species (exceptions

Table 1–1   Classification of Physical Status

Category	Physical Status	Examples
I	Normal healthy patient	Patient presented for elective procedure
II	Patient with mild systemic disease	Skin tumor, fracture without shock
III	Patient with severe but not incapacitating systemic disease	Fever, dehydration, anemia, cachexia, early renal or cardiac disease
IV	Patient with severe life-threatening systemic disease	Uremia, cardiac decompensation, septicemia, emaciation
V	Moribund patient not expected to survive with or without intervention	Profound shock, terminal malignancy, severe trauma
E	E is added to category to designate that anesthesia is being performed on an emergency basis.	

Adapted from the American Society of Anesthesiologists.

being animals in which venipuncture cannot be performed without some level of anesthesia). Blood urea nitrogen (uric acid in avian species) is advised but probably not necessary in most healthy patients. Normal ranges of these values for a variety of species are given in Table 1–3. History and physical examination findings

Table 1–2 Normal Values for Temperature, Pulse Rate, and Respiratory Rate for Several Veterinary Species

Species	Temperature °F	Heart Rate/Minute	Respiratory Rate/Minute
Birds			
Pet birds*	102–105	120–500	10–75
Raptors	102–104	107–310	12–25
Ratites	99–104	60–190	6–12 (resting, mild ambient temperature)
Cat	100.5–102.5	110–200	15–26
Cow	100.5–102.5	60–80	8–20
Dog	101–103	89–140	8–20
Ferret	100–104	200–400	33–36
Goat	101–103	70–135	12–25
Horse	99.5–101.5	25–50	8–12
Llama	99.5–102	60–80	10–30
Rabbit	101.5–104	130–325	30–60
Sheep	102–104	60–90	15–30
Pig	100–103	60–90	10–30
Pot-belly pig	102–103	70–80 (80–100: neonates)	13–18 (25–40: neonates/ juveniles)

*Ranges tend to correlate inversely with the size of the bird.

Table 1-3 Normal (Awake) Ranges for Hematocrit, Total Protein, White Blood Cell Count, and Selected Chemistry Values for Several Veterinary Species

Species	PCV (%)	TP (gm/dl)	WBC × 10³	BUN (mg/dl)	Creatinine (mg/dl)
Birds*					
Pet birds	35–50	2.5–5.0	3.0–12.0	2.3–14.0 mg/dl (Uric acid)	
Raptors	43–49	2.65–5.1	4.6–12	4.5–14 mg/dl (Uric acid)	
Ratites	40–50	2.4–5.3	8–24	1–14 mg/dl (Uric acid)	
Cat	27–45	6.0–7.5	5.5–18	15–31	0.7–1.8
Cow	23–43	6.0–7.5	4–12	7–30	0.6–1.8
Dog	35–54	5.5–7.5	6.5–18	6–30	0.5–1.6
Ferret	48–50	6.0	7.0–9.3	19–27	0.4–0.5
Goat	22–38	6.1–7.4	4–13	12–25	0.7–1.5
Horse	25–48	5.7–7.9	6–12	10–30	0.9–1.8
Llama	25–45	4.9–7.9	8–23	9–33	1.1–3.2
Rabbit	36–48	5.4–7.5	9–11	17–23	0.8–1.8
Sheep	30–50	6.3–7.1	4–12	5–26	0.9–2.0
Pig	30–50	6.0–8.0	6.5–20	8–24	0.8–2.7

Note: These normal values should be used as general guidelines, as variation exists between reference ranges for individual laboratories.

*Wide variation exists among avian species. Values listed are to be used only as general guidelines.

(abnormal organ system function, geriatric patients) will dictate the need for more complete laboratory evaluation including a complete blood count; serum chemistry panel, which should include total CO_2 (metabolic acid-base status) and electrolyte concentrations; and urinalysis. Unprompted extensive laboratory screening has not been found to improve outcome for surgical patients in either human or veterinary medicine. Further diagnostic evaluation, such as thoracic and abdominal radiographs or ultrasonography, echocardiography, and organ specific evaluation (i.e., bile acid assay) should be based on abnormal physical examination and primary blood chemistry findings.

Fasting

In general, patients should be fasted for 6–12 hours prior to induction of anesthesia, with water withheld for variable periods of time to minimize risk of aspiration and regurgitation and to decrease gastrointestinal volume. There is disparity in the literature regarding length of fasting, due largely to personal experience and preference. Table 1–4 lists recommended fasting times for several common domestic species. Slightly longer periods are recommended when prolonged or abdominal surgeries are to be performed. Very young and very small patients should *not* be fasted due to risk of hypoglycemia. Water withholding is unnecessary in most species with the exception being ruminants and camelids (see Table 1–4).

Table 1–4 Recommended Fasting and Water Withholding Times for Several Veterinary Species

Species	Recommended Fasting Time*	Water Restriction**
Birds		
Pet birds	1–3 hr (the smaller the bird, the shorter the fast; >300 gms: *maximum* 10 hr usually is tolerated)	≤1 hr
Raptors	6–12 hr (up to 24 hr in large raptors)	2 hr
Ratites	12–24 hr	2 hr
Cat	6–8 hr	6 hr
Cow	24–48 hr	12–24 hr
Dog	6–8 hr	6 hr
Ferret	4–6 hr	2 hr
Goat	12–24 hr	2–8 hr
Horse	6–12 hr	Not necessary
Llama	12–24 hr	8 hr
Rabbit†	8 hr	Not necessary
Sheep	12–24 hr	2–8 hr
Pig	8–12 hr	Not necessary

Note: Fasting times for many species vary in the literature; as a general rule, the longer the procedure, the longer is the fast.

*Fasting is not recommended for neonates of any species or for very small patients because high metabolic rates and limited glycogen stores cause increased risk for development of hypoglycemia. Fasting should be abbreviated or omitted in animals with diseases that can precipitate hypoglycemia, such as insulinoma and diabetes mellitus.   *(continues)*

Table 1–4 *(Continued)*

**Water deprivation should be eliminated or abbreviated in patients with significant renal disease (unless IV fluids are provided to assure normal hydration preoperatively) or during high ambient environmental temperatures (i.e., ruminants).

†While the practice has been recommended in the literature, fasting of rabbits is considered unnecessary since this species does not vomit and a prolonged fast can promote gastrointestinal stasis.

Record Keeping

Proper patient preparation minimizes but cannot eliminate the risk of anesthesia. Thorough record keeping will encourage vigilant patient monitoring and allow the veterinarian not only to evaluate perianesthetic events retrospectively for future reference but to provide relevant and documented information should litigation occur. The anesthetic record should include animal name and case number, owner name, signalment, weight, physical and laboratory examination results, physical status, procedure performed, all anesthetic agents (premedications, induction agents, maintenance agents) administered including dose (in mg) or concentration (inhalant agents), route and time of administration, duration of anesthesia, supportive measures (i.e., fluid type and rate of administration), a chronologic recording of vital signs, postoperative analgesic agents administered, vital signs recorded during recovery and any complications encountered. Figure 1–1 provides an example of an anesthetic record to facilitate complete record keeping.

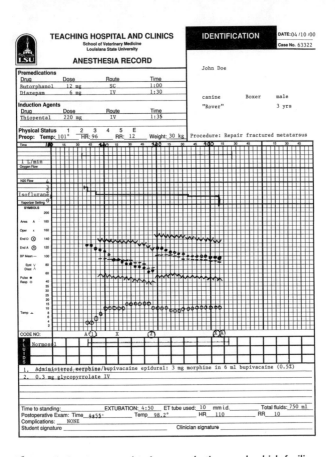

Figure 1-1 An example of an anesthetic record, which facilitates sequential recording of vital signs and summarizes drugs administered and events occurring during the anesthetic period.

2

Pharmacology and Application of Parenteral Anesthetic Agents

A plethora of injectable agents are available in veterinary practice to fulfill the need for premedication, induction, maintenance, and postoperative analgesia; to alleviate anxiety and motor activity (chemical restraint); and to provide profound muscle relaxation (neuromuscular blocking agents) when indicated. While some agents, such as the dissociative drugs, serve multiple roles (premedication, induction, and maintenance), parenteral drugs are summarized according to primary effects and briefly described in Table 2–1. The "ideal" anesthetic agent is described in Table 2–2. Because no drug available today possesses all the "ideal" qualities, anesthetic selection is a compromise based on the patient, the procedure, and the available agents, equipment, and expertise. Inhalation agents come *closest* to possessing the majority of qualities described for an "ideal" anesthetic agent and will be discussed in Chapter 4.

Premedication agents are used to aid in animal restraint (calming effect), reduce anxiety, provide analgesia, provide muscle relaxation, decrease the requirements for potentially more dangerous drugs used for induction and maintenance, promote smooth transition from consciousness to unconsciousness and vice versa during the induction and recovery periods, respectively, and minimize autonomic reflex activity. Induction agents are used to provide a smooth transition from consciousness to unconsciousness, which facilitates intubation and transition to the maintenance protocol. *Some* agents used for induction also are useful, as repeat boluses or constant rate infusion, for maintenance of anesthesia (see Table 2–1). Other drugs (adjunct agents, Table 2–1) serve a variety of roles including sparing the more cardiorespiratory depressing drugs used for induction and maintenance and muscle relaxation.

The following alphabetical list (by chemical name) summarizes drugs that might be used in veterinary anesthesia (MOA is mechanism of action; DOA is duration of action, these numbers are only guidelines as DOA is influenced significantly by concurrently administered drugs and individual patient status). Route of administration for every agent is listed in parentheses after DOA and includes intravenous (IV), intramuscular (IM), subcutaneous (SC), and per os (PO). In general, the onset of effect occurs within 5 minutes for drugs administered intravenously. When drugs are administered intramuscularly, onset of effect is in 15 minutes; subcutaneous administration requires a slightly longer time to take effect (20–30 minutes). Common tradenames (USA; UK* *or* USA and UK**) for some of the agents have been listed in parentheses after the chemical name. Drug dosages are listed in Appendix 1 and in those chapters discussing protocols for individual animal species.

Drug:	**Aceapromazine (Promace; Acetylpromazine*)**
Class:	Phenothiazine tranquilizer (major)
MOA:	Antiadrenergic, anticholinergic, antihistaminic, antidopaminergic
DOA:	Dose dependent; 2–3 hr (prolonged in hepatic-compromised, geriatric, and pediatric patients); (IV, IM, SC, PO)
Effect:	Calming effect; decreased motor activity; antiemetic; *no analgesia*
Adverse:	Hypotension, penile paralysis (equine), decreased seizure threshold, prolonged duration with liver disease; anecdotal reports of profound respiratory and cardiovascular depression in Boxers
Approved:	Horses, cats, dogs

Drug: **Alfentanil (Alfenta; Rapifen*):** Schedule II

Class: Opioid agonist

MOA: Activates μ opioid receptors

DOA: <30 minutes; used as constant rate infusion; (IV)

Effect: Analgesia, sedation

Adverse: Respiratory depression, bradycardia, excitement in some species

Approved: None; rarely used in veterinary medicine

Drug: **Atipamezole (Antisedan)**

Class: Alpha$_2$ receptor antagonist

MOA: Blocks alpha$_1$ and alpha$_2$ receptors

DOA: >120 minutes; (IM)

Effect: Reverses effects of alpha$_2$ agonists

Adverse: Excitement, tremors, salivation, vomiting, diarrhea

Approved: Dogs

Drug: **Atracurium (Tracrium**)**

Class: Competitive nondepolarizing neuromuscular blocking agent

MOA: Competitive blockade of acetylcholine receptors at neuromuscular junction

DOA: <30 minutes (undergoes Hofmann elimination: spontaneous nonenzymatic degradation at body pH; also metabolized by esterases); (IV)

Effect: Reversible skeletal muscle relaxation

Adverse: Respiratory paralysis (must support respiration), minimal cardiovascular effects, may cause histamine release

Approved: None

Drug: **Atropine**

Class: Anticholinergic

MOA: Competitive blockade of muscarinic receptors

DOA: 60–90 min (some species variation); (IV, IM, SC)

Effect: Parasympatholytic: increased heart rate, decreased salivation/secretions, dilated pupils; gastrointestinal stasis, increases physiologic dead space (bronchodilation)

Adverse: Tachycardia, arrhythmias, colic (equine)

Approved: Dogs, cats, cattle, horses, sheep

Drug: **Azaperone (Stresnil**)**

Class: Butyrophenone tranquilizer (major)

MOA: Antiadrenergic, anticholinergic, antihistaminic, antidopaminergic

DOA: 2–4 hr; (IV, IM)

Effect: Calming effect; decreased motor activity; antiemetic; *no analgesia*

Adverse: Extrapyramidal effects (tremors, rigidity) are more common compared to acepromazine; personality change possible; hypotension

Approved: Swine

Drug: **Bupivacaine (Marcaine**): 0.5%**

Class: Local anesthetic agent (amide)

MOA: Blocks nerve transmission by blocking Na channel and preventing excitation-conduction process

DOA: 4–6 hr; (epidural, local infiltration)

Effect: Reversible prevention of nerve transmission; thus motor, sensory, and autonomic function is temporarily inhibited

Adverse: CNS excitation, seizures, respiratory paralysis, hypotension, hypothermia, ventricular arrhythmias

Approved: None

Drug: **Buprenorphine (Buprenex; Temgesic*; Vetergesic*):** Schedule V

Class: Opioid partial agonist

MOA: Activates opioid receptors in brain and spinal cord

DOA: 6–12 hr; (IV, IM, SC)

Effect: Analgesia; minimal sedation

Adverse: Respiratory depression (less than with pure opioid agonists), bradycardia, flatulence, defecation, hypothermia; may be more difficult to reverse due to high receptor affinity

Approved: None

Drug: **Butorphanol (Torbugesic**; Torbutrol**):** Schedule IV

Class: Opioid agonist/antagonist

MOA: Activates (κ) and blocks (μ) opioid receptors in brain and spinal cord

DOA: 1–2 hr; (IV, IM, SC, PO)

Effect: Analgesia, sedation

Adverse: Respiratory depression (less than with pure opioids), bradycardia, flatulence, defecation, hypothermia

Approved: Horses, dogs

Drug: **Carfentanil (Wildnil):** Schedule II (requires DEA special user's permit)

Class: Opioid agonist

MOA: Activates opioid μ receptors

DOA: Prolonged if not reversed; (IM)

Effect:	Analgesia, sedation, immobilization
Adverse:	Hypoventilation, excitement (some species), hypothermia, muscle fasciculations
Approved:	Animal use only, reserved for use in immobilization of wildlife and exotic species

Drug:	**Chloral hydrate:** Schedule IV
Class:	Sedative-hypnotic
MOA:	CNS depression is due to active metabolites
DOA:	Dose dependent: <2 hr for sedative dosages; (IV, PO)
Effect:	Sedation at low doses; general anesthetic at high doses; poor analgesic effects
Adverse:	Minimal at sedative dosages; anesthetic doses have high incidence of cardiopulmonary arrest
Approved:	None; once available in combination with pentobarbital and magnesium sulfate for use in large animals

Drug:	**cis-Atracurium (Nimbex)**
Class:	Competitive nondepolarizing neuromuscular blocking agent

MOA: Competitive blockade of acetylcholine receptors of neuromuscular junction

DOA: <20–30 min (undergoes Hofmann elimination: spontaneous nonenzymatic degradation at body pH); (IV)

Effect: Reversible skeletal muscle relaxation

Adverse: Respiratory paralysis (must control respiration), minimal cardiovascular effects

Approved: None

Drug: **Desflurane (Suprane)**

Class: Methyl ether inhalation agent

MOA: Reversible depression of central nervous system

DOA: Not applicable

Effect: Unconsciousness, analgesia, muscle relaxation

Adverse: Dose-dependent cardiopulmonary depression (slightly less than other inhalation agents at equivalent MAC concentrations)

Approved: None

Drug: **Detomidine (Dormosedan)**

Class: Alpha$_2$ agonist

MOA: Activates CNS alpha$_2$ receptors, which inhibit neurotransmitter release in brain

DOA: Dose dependent; 75–120 min; (IV, IM)

Effect: Sedation, analgesia, muscle relaxation

Adverse: Bradycardia, conduction disturbances, hypotension, respiratory depression, hypoxia

Approved: Horses

Drug: **Diazepam (Valium**):** Schedule IV

Class: Benzodiazepine tranquilizer (minor)

MOA: Activates CNS benzodiazepine receptors, which increase inhibitory neurotransmitters (i.e., GABA, glycine)

DOA: <3 hr; (IV, IM, PO)

Effect: Mild sedation, muscle relaxation, enhances effect of concurrently used agents

Adverse: Excitement in some species (horses, dogs), hepatoxicity has been reported with PO administration in cats

Approved: Dog

Drug: **Diprenorphine (Revivon*, M$_{50-50}$)**

Class: Opioid agonist/antagonist

MOA: Blocks opioid receptors

DOA: Short (renarcotization following reversal of potent opioids has been reported); (IV, IM)

Effect:	Used to antagonize etorphine
Adverse:	Opioid sedation and respiratory depression may persist with overdose
Approved:	Animal use only, for reversal of etorphine in wildlife and exotic species

Drug:	**Edrophonium (Tensilon)**
Class:	Acetylcholinesterase inhibitor
MOA:	Inhibits acetylcholinesterase and allows accumulation of ACh, enhances ACh release, induces repetitive firing of the motor nerve terminal
DOA:	Onset of action is rapid (1–2 min); duration relatively short; (IV)
Effect:	Antagonize nondepolarizing neuromuscular blockers to restore neuromuscular transmission
Adverse:	Parasympathetic stimulation: bradycardia, airway constriction, increased secretions
Approved:	None

Drug:	**Enflurane (Ethrane**): an isomer of isoflurane**
Class:	Methyl ether: inhalation agent
MOA:	Reversible depression of central nervous system

DOA: Not applicable

Effect: Unconsciousness, muscle relaxation

Adverse: Dose-dependent cardiac and respiratory depression

Approved: None

Drug: **Etomidate (Amidate; Hypnomidate*)**

Class: Imidazole

MOA: Nonbarbiturate sedative-hypnotic

DOA: <10 min; (IV)

Effect: Rapid loss of consciousness of short duration, minimal cardiopulmonary depression

Adverse: Pain on injection, myoclonus, vomiting (minimized with premedication); depression of adrenal function

Approved: None

Drug: **Etorphine (M-99):** Schedule II

Class: Opioid agonist

MOA: Activates μ opioid receptors

DOA: <2 hr; (IV, IM)

Effect: Sedation, analgesia, immobilization, 80–1,000 times as potent as morphine

Adverse: *Profound* respiratory depression, bradycardia, hypertension

Approved: Animal use only: exotic animal immobilization

Drug: **Fentanyl (Sublimaze**):** Schedule II

Class: Opioid agonist

MOA: Activates μ opioid receptors

DOA: <1 hr; used as constant rate infusion (IV) or transdermal patch

Effect: Analgesia, sedation, 75–125 times as potent as morphine

Adverse: Respiratory depression, bradycardia, excitement in some species

Approved: None

Drug: **Flumazenil (Romazicon)**

Class: Benzodiazepine receptor antagonist

MOA: Competes with benzodiazepines for receptor

DOA: 2–3 hr; (IV)

Effect: Specific reversal of benzodiazepine tranquilizers

Adverse: Rare

Approved: None

Drug: **Gallamine (Flaxedil**):** currently not available commercially

Class: Nondepolarizing neuromuscular blocker

MOA: Competitive blockade of acetylcholine receptors of neuromuscular junction; prevents muscle contraction

DOA: <30 min; (IV)

Effect: Reversible skeletal muscle relaxation

Adverse: Respiratory paralysis, tachycardia, hypertension

Approved: None (has been used in reptiles for immobilization)

Drug: **Glycopyrrolate (Robinul)**

Class: Anticholinergic

MOA: Blocks effect of acetylcholine at muscarinic receptors

DOA: 2–4 hr; (IV, IM, SC)

Effect: Parasympatholytic: increased heart rate, decreased respiratory secretions, increases physiologic dead space (bronchodilation), does not cross placental or blood-brain barrier

Adverse: Ileus, sinus tachycardia

Approved: Dog, cat

Drug: **Guaifenesin (Guailaxin; Glycerol guaiacolate)**

Class: Central-acting muscle relaxant

MOA: Depresses internuncial neuron transmission; central-acting muscle relaxant

DOA: Dose dependent; 30 min; (IV)

Effect: Muscle relaxation, sedation

Adverse: Very safe although overdose can occur, which manifests as forelimb rigidity followed by respiratory paralysis

Approved: Horses

Drug: **Halothane (Fluothane**)**

Class: Fluorinated hydrocarbon inhalation anesthetic

MOA: Reversible depression of central nervous system

DOA: Not applicable

Effect: Unconsciousness, muscle relaxation

Adverse: Dose-dependent cardiopulmonary depression, ventricular arrhythmias

Approved: Dogs, cats, nonfood animals

Drug: **Isoflurane (Aerrane, Isoflo; Forane**)**

Class: Methyl ether inhalation anesthetic

MOA: Reversible depression of central nervous system

DOA: Not applicable

Effect: Unconsciousness, muscle relaxation

Adverse: Dose-dependent cardiopulmonary depression (relatively less than halothane)

Approved: Horses, dogs

Drug: **Ketamine (Ketaset; Ketalar*; Vetalar**)**

Class: Dissociative agent

MOA: Depresses thalamoneocortical system; activates limbic system; analgesic effects are associated with opioid (agonist) and N-methyl-D-aspartate receptor (antagonist) interaction

DOA: Dose and species dependent; 15–60 min; (IV, IM)

Effect: Catalepsy, superficial analgesia, poor visual analgesia, amnesia, immobility

Adverse: Muscle rigidity, seizures, increased secretions, negative inotropic agent but central catecholamine release causes increased ABP and HR, increased ocular and intracranial pressure

Approved: Cats, primates

Drug: **Lidocaine (Xylocaine**): 2.0%**

Class: Local anesthetic agent (amide)

MOA: Blocks sodium influx and thus prevents nerve depolarization and conduction

DOA: 90–200 min; (epidural, local infiltration)

Effect: Blocks pain, motor, and sympathetic fibers; also used IV to treat ventricular arrhythmias

Adverse: Hypotension due to vasodilation; respiratory arrest is possible when given epidurally; seizures at high doses

Approved: None

Drug: **Medetomidine (Dormitor)**

Class: Alpha$_2$ agonist

MOA: Activates CNS alpha$_2$ receptors, which inhibit neurotransmitter release in brain

DOA: Dose and species dependent; 60–120 min; (IV, IM, SC)

Effect: Sedation, analgesia, muscle relaxation

Adverse: Bradycardia, conduction disturbances, hypotension, respiratory depression, hypoxia

Approved: Dogs

Drug: **Meperidine (Demerol; Pethidine*):** Schedule II

Class: Opioid agonist

MOA: Activates µ receptors in CNS and other organs

DOA: <2 hr; (IM, SC)

Effect: Analgesia, sedation, increases venous capacitance

Adverse: Respiratory depression, flatulence, constipation, bradycardia, can cause histamine release with rapid IV injection, excitement possible in cats, horses

Approved: None

Drug: **Mepivicaine (Carbocaine-V): 1–2%**

Class: Local anesthetic agent (amide)

MOA: Blocks sodium influx and thus prevents nerve depolarization and conduction

DOA: 120–240 min; (epidural, local infiltration)

Effect: Blocks pain, motor and sympathetic fibers

Adverse: Hypotension due to vasodilation and respiratory arrest are possible when given epidurally; seizures and cardiotoxicity with overdose

Approved: None

Drug: **Methohexital (Brevital; Brevane; Brietal*):** Schedule IV

Class: Ultrashort-acting oxybarbiturate

MOA: Sedative-hypnotic; CNS depression by action on barbiturate receptors

DOA:	<15 min; (IV)
Effect:	Sedation to unconsciousness (dose dependent)
Adverse:	Respiratory depression (apnea), myocardial depression, excitement, muscle tremors, seizures during recovery
Approved:	None

Drug:	**Methoxyflurane (Metofane**; Penthrane)**
Class:	Methyl ether inhalation anesthetic
MOA:	Reversible depression of central nervous system
DOA:	Not applicable
Effect:	Unconsciousness, analgesia, muscle relaxation
Adverse:	Dose-dependent cardiopulmonary depression; *prolonged* recovery; renal toxicity due to metabolites
Approved:	Small and large animals, birds

Drug:	**Midazolam (Versed; Hypnovel*):** Schedule IV
Class:	Benzodiazepine tranquilizer (minor)
MOA:	Activates CNS benzodiazepine receptors, which increase inhibitory neurotransmittors (i.e., GABA, glycine)

DOA:	<2 hr (duration is slightly less than diazepam); (IV, IM, SC)
Effect:	Mild sedation, muscle relaxation; works well IV or IM
Adverse:	Excitement in some species, respiratory depression
Approved:	None

Drug:	**Morphine (Duromorph**):** Schedule II
Class:	Opioid agonist
MOA:	Activates μ opioid receptors in CNS and other organs
DOA:	4 hr; (IM, SC, PO)
Effect:	Analgesia, sedation, alleviates pulmonary edema by increasing venous capacitance; provides 10–24 hr of analgesia as far forward as the thoracic limbs when administered epidurally.
Adverse:	Respiratory depression, flatulence, constipation, histamine release with IV administration; excitement possible in horses and cats
Approved:	None

Drug:	**Nalbuphine (Nubain)**
Class:	Opioid agonist/antagonist

MOA:	Antagonizes μ receptor, activates kappa receptors
DOA:	2–3 hr; (IV, IM, SC)
Effect:	Analgesia, sedation
Adverse:	Minimal respiratory depression
Approved:	None

Drug:	**Nalmefene (Revex)**
Class:	Opioid antagonist
MOA:	Antagonizes all opioid receptors
DOA:	Longer acting than naloxone; (IV, IM, SC)
Effect:	Reverses effects of opioid agonists, including respiratory depression and analgesia
Adverse:	Stimulates sympathetic nervous system; potential for cardiac arrhythmias
Approved:	None

Drug:	**Naloxone (Narcan**)**
Class:	Opioid antagonist
MOA:	Antagonizes all opioid receptors
DOA:	30–45 min; (IV, IM, SC)
Effect:	Reverses the effects of opioid agonists, including respiratory depression and

analgesia; has been used in the treatment of hemorrhagic shock

Adverse: Stimulates sympathetic nervous system: potential for cardiac arrhythmias

Approved: None

Drug: **Naltrexone (Trexonil)**

Class: Opioid antagonist

MOA: Antagonizes all opioid receptors

DOA: Longer acting than naloxone; (IV, IM, SC)

Effect: Reverses the effects of opioid agonists, including respiratory depression and analgesia; available as an oral preparation for humans

Adverse: Stimulates sympathetic nervous system: potential for cardiac arrhythmias

Approved: Used for reversal of carfentanil in exotic species

Drug: **Neostigmine (Prostigmine; Stiglyn)**

Class: Acetylcholinesterase inhibitor

MOA: Inhibits acetylcholinesterase and allows accumulation of ACh, enhances ACh release, induces repetitive firing of the motor nerve terminal

DOA:	Onset of action is 7–10 min; duration of action is relatively short; (IV)
Effect:	Antagonize nondepolarizing neuromuscular blockers to restore neuromuscular transmission, onset of action is rapid
Adverse:	Parasympathetic stimulation including bradycardia, airway constriction, increased secretions
Approved:	None

Drug:	**Oxymorphone (Numorphan):** Schedule II
Class:	Opioid agonist
MOA:	Activates μ receptors
DOA:	2–6 hr; (IV, IM, SC)
Effect:	Analgesia, sedation
Adverse:	Respiratory depression, bradycardia, excitement in some species
Approved:	Dogs, cats

Drug:	**Pancuronium (Pavulon******)**
Class:	Competitive nondepolarizing neuromuscular blocker
DOA:	30–45 min; (IV)
MOA:	Competitive blockade of acetylcholine receptors of neuromuscular junction

Effect: Reversible skeletal muscle paralysis

Adverse: Respiratory paralysis (must control ventilation), minimal cardiovascular effects although may cause transient tachycardia; prolonged effect in renal- and hepatic-compromised patients

Approved: None

Drug: **Pentazocine (Talwin):** Schedule IV

Class: Opioid agonist/antagonist

MOA: Activates (κ) and blocks (μ) opioid receptors in brain and spinal cord: low potency

DOA: <2 hr; (IM, SC)

Effect: Analgesia, sedation; 0.1–0.3 times potency of morphine

Adverse: Respiratory depression (less than with pure opioids), bradycardia, flatulence, defecation, hypothermia

Approved: Horses, dogs

Drug: **Pentobarbital (Nembutal; Beuthanasia-D):** Schedule II

Class: Short-acting oxybarbiturate

MOA: Sedative-hypnotic; CNS depression by action on barbiturate receptors

DOA: Species and dose dependent; <1.5 hr; (IV, PO)

Effect: Sedation to unconsciousness

Adverse: CNS/respiratory depression (apnea), myocardial depression, leukopenia, splenic engorgement, excitement (stage II) due to inadequate quantity or rate of dosing

Approved: Dogs

Drug: **Phenobarbital:** Schedule IV

Class: Long-acting oxybarbiturate; routes include IV and PO

MOA: Sedative/hypnotic; CNS depression by action on barbiturate receptors

DOA: Dose dependent; 12–24 hr; (IV, PO)

Effect: Sedation to unconsciousness (dose dependent); used to control seizures: (16 mg/kg IV, 2–4 mg/kg PO BID (small animal); 2–10 mg/kg IV/PO every 8–12 hr (equine)

Adverse: CNS/respiratory depression (apnea), myocardial depression, polyuria/polydipsia/polyphagia

Approved: None

Drug: **Procaine (Novocaine)**

Class: Local anesthetic (ester linked)

MOA: Blocks sodium influx and thus prevents nerve depolarization and conduction

DOA: 60–90 min; (local infiltration)

Effect: Blocks pain, motor, and sympathetic fibers

Adverse: May cause allergic reaction

Approved: None

Drug: **Propofol (Rapinovet**)**

Class: Alkyl phenol structure

MOA: Sedative/hypnotic: CNS depression by enhancing GABA activity in the brain and decreasing cerebral metabolic rate

DOA: <15 min; (IV)

Effect: Sedation to unconsciousness depending on dosage; muscle relaxation

Adverse: Respiratory depression (*apnea*) especially if administered rapidly, myocardial depression, hypotension, Heinz body formation (oxidative injury) in cats when given repeatedly due to phenolic structure

Approved: Dogs

Drug:　　　**Pyridostigmine (Regonol)**

Class:　　Acetylcholinesterase inhibitor

MOA:　　Inhibit acetylcholinesterase and allow accumulation of ACh, enhance ACh release, induce repetitive firing of the motor nerve terminal

DOA:　　Onset of action is 12–16 min and duration 40% longer than neostigmine and edrophonium; (IV)

Effect:　　Antagonize nondepolarizing neuromuscular blockers to restore neuromuscular transmission

Adverse:　　Parasympathetic stimulation, including bradycardia, airway constriction, increased secretions

Approved: None

Drug:　　　**Romifidine (Sedivet*)**

Class:　　Alpha$_2$ agonist

MOA:　　Activates CNS alpha$_2$ receptors, which inhibit neurotransmitter release in brain

DOA:　　Dose dependent; >120 min; (IV, IM, SC)

Effect:　　Sedation, analgesia, muscle relaxation

Adverse:　　Bradycardia, conduction disturbances, hypotension, respiratory depression, hypoxia

Approved: Not currently approved in the United States, but studies have been published for dosages in dogs and horses

Drug: **Sevoflurane (Ultrane)**

Class: Methyl ether inhalation agent

MOA: Reversible depression of central nervous system

DOA: Not applicable

Effect: Unconsciousness, muscle relaxation

Adverse: Dose-dependent cardiopulmonary depression (similar to isoflurane)

Approved: None

Drug: **Succinylcholine (Anectine**; Sucostrin; Scoline*)**

Class: Depolarizing noncompetitive neuromuscular blocker

MOA: Depolarizes nicotinic receptors on muscle motor end plate and prevents neuromuscular transmission.

DOA: <15 min; (IV)

Effect: Nonreversible (short-duration) skeletal muscle paralysis

Adverse: Respiratory paralysis (necessary equipment to provide mechanical ventilation should be available if this drug is used);

prolonged effect with hepatic-compromising diseases due to dependency on metabolism by the liver-derived enzyme, pseudocholinesterase; muscle fasciculations; hyperkalemia; known trigger of malignant hyperthermia

Approved: None

Drug:	**Sufentanil (Sufenta):** Schedule II
Class:	Opioid agonist
MOA:	Activates μ opioid receptors
DOA:	<1 hr; used as constant rate infusion; (IV)
Effect:	Analgesia, sedation
Adverse:	Respiratory depression, bradycardia, muscle twitching
Approved:	None; rarely used in veterinary medicine

Drug:	**Thiopental (Pentothal; Intraval*):** Schedule III
Class:	Ultrashort-acting thiobarbiturate
MOA:	Sedative/hypnotic; CNS depression by action on barbiturate receptors
DOA:	<15 min; (IV)
Effect:	Sedation to unconsciousness (dose dependent), stage II delerium can occur with inadequate or perivascular dosages

Adverse:	Respiratory depression (apnea), myocardial depression, cardiac arrhythmias
Approved:	Dogs

Drug:	**Tiletamine; Zolazepam (Telazol):** Schedule III
Class:	Dissociative agent combined with benzodiazepine
MOA:	Tiletamine: depresses thalamoneocortical system; activates limbic system; analgesic effects are associated with opioid (agonist) and N-methyl-D-aspartate receptor (antagonist) interaction; zolazepam acts on benzodiazepine receptors
DOA:	Dose and species dependent; 20–80 min; (IM, IV)
Effect:	Catalepsy, superficial analgesia, amnesia, immobility, muscle relaxation
Adverse:	Increased secretions, muscle rigidity in some species, negative inotrope but central catecholamine release promotes increased BP and HR, increased ocular and intracranial pressure
Approved:	Cats, dogs

Drug:	**Tolazoline (Tolazine)**
Class:	Alpha$_1$ and alpha$_2$ receptor antagonist

MOA: Occupies and antagonizes alpha$_2$ receptors (least specific for the alpha$_2$ receptor)

DOA: 2 hr; (IV, IM)

Effect: Reverses effects of alpha$_2$ agonists

Adverse: Hypotension with rapid injection due to vasodilatory effect, excitement, tremors, salivation, tachypnea

Approved: Horses

Drug: **Tubocurarine (Curare)**

Class: Competitive nondepolarizing neuromuscular blocker

MOA: Competitive blockade of acetylcholine receptors of neuromuscular junction

DOA: <30 min; (IV)

Effect: Reversible skeletal muscle relaxation

Adverse: Respiratory paralysis (must control respiration), causes histamine release that results in hypotension and bronchoconstriction

Approved: None

Drug: **Vecuronium (Norcuron)**

Class: Competitive nondepolarizing neuromuscular blocker

MOA: Competitive blockade of acetylcholine
            receptors of neuromuscular junction

DOA: <30 min; (IV)

Effect: Reversible skeletal muscle relaxation

Adverse: Respiratory paralysis (must control respi-
            ration), minimal cardiovascular effects;
            significant hepatic dysfunction will pro-
            long effect

Approved: None

Drug: **Xylazine (Rompun**; Ansed)**

Class: Alpha$_2$ agonist

MOA: Activates CNS alpha$_2$ receptors, which
            inhibit neurotransmitter release in brain

DOA: Dose and species dependent; 15–30 min
            (analgesia); 1–2 hr (sedation); (IV, IM,
            SC)

Effect: Sedation, analgesia, muscle relaxation

Adverse: Bradycardia, conduction disturbances,
            hypotension, respiratory depression,
            hypoxia

Approved: Horses (10% formulation); dogs and cats
            (2% formulation); deer and elk

Drug:	**Yohimbine (Yobine)**
Class:	Alpha$_2$ antagonist
MOA:	Blocks alpha$_2$ receptors; also has antiserotonin activity
DOA:	<1 hr; (IV, IM)
Effect:	Reverses effects of alpha$_2$ agonists
Adverse:	Hypotension with rapid injection due to vasodilatory effect, excitement, tremors, salivation, tachypnea
Approved:	Dogs

Table 2–1   Categories and Major Effects of Injectable Anesthetic Agents Used in Veterinary Medicine (text has specific agent information)

Use/Category	Effects/Comments
Premedications	
Anticholinergics	Decrease secretions, prevent bradycardia
Atropine	
Glycopyrrolate	
Tranquilizers	Alleviate anxiety and decrease motor activity; provide *no* analgesia, synergize activity of other agents; promote muscle relaxation
Major tranquilizers:	
Acepromazine (phenothiazine)	Use is relatively common in all species
Azaperone (butyrophenone)	Use is predominantly in swine and some exotic species
Minor tranquilizers:	
Diazepam (benzodiazepine)	Minimal sedation unless combined with opioid or alpha$_2$ agonist
Midazolam	More rapid onset of effect and not painful when given IM or

(benzodiazepine)	SC (compared to diazepam, which is recommended for IV use only)
Benzodiazepine antagonist Flumazenil	Specific reversal agent for benzodiazepines
Alpha₂ agonists	Provide analgesia, sedation, and muscle relaxation; cardiovascular effects are profound (conduction disturbances, hypotension) but usually well-tolerated in healthy patients; significant sparing effect when used prior to inhalant anesthesia
Xylazine	Shortest duration of effect; $\alpha_2{:}\alpha_1$ selectivity binding ratio = 160
Detomidine	Longest duration of effect; $\alpha_2{:}\alpha_1$ selectivity binding ratio = 260
Medetomidine	Greatest $\alpha_2{:}\alpha_1$ selectivity binding ratio = 1620
Romifidine	Not currently approved for use in United States; $\alpha_2{:}\alpha_1$ selectivity binding ratio = 340
Alpha₂ antagonists	Specific reversal agents for alpha₂ agonists; may promote hypotension through vasodilatory effects especially when administered rapidly IV
Yohimbine	$\alpha_2{:}\alpha_1$ selectivity binding ratio = 40

(continues)

Table 2–1   *(Continued)*

Use/Category	Effects/Comments
Tolazoline	Nonspecific antagonist of α_1 and α_2 receptors
Atipamezole	$\alpha_2 : \alpha_1$ selectivity binding ratio = 8526
Opioids	Provide analgesia and sedation (degree of effects vary with agent); used for preemptive and postoperative analgesia. (Analgesic potencies relative to morphine [1] are listed in parentheses for each agent.)
Opioid (μ) agonists:	Major side effect is respiratory depression; greatest potential for abuse
Morphine	(1)
Meperidine	(0.5)
Hydromorphone	(5)
Oxymorphone	(8–10)
Fentanyl	(75–125)
Alfentanil	(20–75)
Sufentanil	(600–1000)
Carfentanil	(10,000)
Etorphine	(80–1000)

Partial μ agonist:

Buprenorphine — Less respiratory depression (25–50)

Opioid agonist (κ)/antagonists (μ):

Butorphanol — Less respiratory depression compared to μ agonists

Commonly used in veterinary medicine; moderate analgesia; may be used to reverse μ agonists; (2–5)

Nalbuphine — Not scheduled but minimally effective as an analgesic agent; may be used to reverse μ agonists; (0.5)

Pentazocine — (0.1)

Nalorphine — Used for antagonist effect, rarely used clinically

Diprenorphine — Used for antagonist effect; short duration of action may allow "renarcotization" after reversal

Opioid antagonists:

Used "to effect" to reverse opioid agonists and agonist/antagonists

Naloxone — Short duration of action may allow "renarcotization" after reversal

Naltrexone

Nalmefene

Dissociative agents — Dose-dependent effect provides quieting and immobilization at low doses and general anesthesia at higher dosages, somatic analgesia; poor visceral analgesia

(continues)

Table 2–1 (Continued)

Use/Category	Effects/Comments
Ketamine	
Tiletamine (Telazol™)	Commercial product combined with zolazepam in 1:1 (mg) ratio
Chloral hydrate	Sedative/hypnotic: used for large animal sedation; no longer used as large animal general anesthetic due to narrow safety margin and prolonged recoveries; effective IV, PO, rectally

Induction/maintenance agents

Barbiturates	Short and ultrashort-acting; high pH makes them irritating to tissues
Pentobarbital	Short-acting oxybarbiturate; recovery >6–24 hr; rarely used for clinical anesthesia due to availability of agents with shorter duration of effect
Methohexital	Ultrashort-acting oxybarbiturate (rapidly metabolized); not commonly used
Thiopental	Ultrashort-acting thiobarbiturate (rapidly redistributed): risk of rough, prolonged recovery if used as repeated bolus or in presence of hepatic disease; common use in veterinary practice

Dissociative agents	See earlier; while metabolism is relatively rapid, repeat dosages of dissociatives will contribute to rough, prolonged recoveries (especially tiletamine)
Propofol	Produces rapid loss of consciousness; recovery is fast due to rapid metabolism, making it useful for induction *and* maintenance
Etomidate	Produces rapid loss of consciousness; recovery is fast due to rapid metabolism, making it useful for induction *and* maintenance
Adjunct agents	
Glyceryl guaiacolate (guaifenesin)	Central-acting muscle relaxant used in large animals to reduce requirements of induction and maintenance agents; 5 and 10% (horses only) solutions—*10% solution causes hemolysis in species other than horses*
Neuromuscular blocking agents	Act at neuromuscular junction to block neurotransmission, resulting in muscle paralysis; ventilatory support is required; useful adjunct for ocular, orthopedic, and abdominal procedures and for patients that resist mechanical ventilation; *sparing effect on concurrently used drugs; no inherent analgesic effects*

(continues)

Table 2-1 (Continued)

Use/Category	Effects/Comments
Nondepolarizing competitive agents:	Competitive (reversible) interference with acetylcholine at postsynaptic muscle membrane; many agents currently available with variable duration of action, cardiovascular effects, ability to induce histamine release, duration and onset of effect and cost (text descriptions are given only for those with current or historical, and relatively common, use in veterinary medicine)
Turbocuraine	Use is largely reserved for research
Gallamine	Use is largely reserved for research and some exotic species
Pancuronium	Relatively long duration of effect
Vecuronium	Intermediate duration of effect
Atracurium	Short duration of effect
cis-Atracurium	Short duration of effect
Mivacurium	Short duration of effect
Rocuronium	Intermediate duration of effect
Doxacurium	Relatively long duration of effect

Depolarizing noncompetitive agents:	Nonreversible depolarization of postsynaptic muscle membrane
Succinylcholine	Ultrashort acting, rapid onset; side effects preclude routine use
Acetylcholinesterase inhibitors:	Reverse competitive NMBs by allowing acetylcholine to accumulate at synaptic cleft and restore normal muscle function; side effects are associated with stimulation of muscarinic receptors and prevented by prior administration of an anticholinergic agent
Edrophonium Neostigmine Pyridostigmine	

Table 2–2 Properties of an "Ideal" Anesthetic Agent

1. Does not require metabolism for termination of action and elimination (reversible or respiratory elimination).
2. Permits rapid and easily controlled induction, changes in anesthetic depth and recovery.
3. Is not irritating to any tissue.
4. Does not depress cardiopulmonary function.
5. Produces adequate muscle relaxation and analgesia for surgical procedures.
6. Is compatible with other drugs.
7. Is nontoxic to the patient and humans.
8. Is inexpensive, stable, and noninflammable.
9. Requires no special equipment for administration.

3

Local/Regional Anesthetic Techniques

Local and regional anesthesia always has been an integral part of large animal practice for economic and practical reasons. The availability and convenience of a variety of general anesthesia options minimized the need to apply these agents in small animals. However, with the ever-increasing awareness of pain management in all veterinary species, local and regional techniques are gaining popularity in small animal practice. Application of local and regional agents in animals undergoing general anesthesia will provide preemptive analgesia and spare anesthetic requirements. While historically such techniques have been associated with the local anesthetic agents, other drugs, including opioids, alpha$_2$ agonists, and ketamine have been reported to possess analgesic properties when applied by these routes. This chapter discusses mainly the application of local anesthetic agents used to produce local and regional anesthesia (complete loss of sensation to a body part or region) but also includes dosage and application of the alpha$_2$ agonists. Clinical application of opioids to produce regional analgesia (loss of sensitivity to pain) is discussed in Chapter 8 ("Pain Management").

Local anesthetic agents reversibly block action potentials along nerve axons by interference with voltage-gated sodium channels. Two classes (based on the intermediate chain of the molecule), the esters and the amides (Table 3–1), determine drug biotransformation. Esters are readily hydrolyzed in the blood by plasma cholinesterase made in the liver, while amides require biotransformation by liver microsomal enzymes. Even though lidocaine is well-known for its usefulness intravenously to treat cardiac ventricular arrhythmias, it and local anesthetic agents have several potential adverse effects, including formation of cardiac arrhythmias (Table 3–2). These adverse effects are minimized when accidental intravenous injection is avoided and dosages remain within recommended maximum safe limits.

The time to effect, potency, and duration of effect depend on the agent's physical and chemical properties (see Table 3–1). Lipid solubility influences intrinsic potency and protein binding is probably the primary determinant of duration. The dissociation constant (pKa) is thought to determine the speed of action. The

Table 3–1 Properties of Selected Local Anesthetic Agents Used in Veterinary Medicine

Agent (Trade Name)	Class	Potency*	Lipid Solubility	pKa	Protein Binding	Onset of Effect	Duration (min)
Procaine (Novocaine)	Ester	—	1	8.9	6%	Slow	60–90
Chloroprocaine (Nesacaine)	Ester	1	1	9.1	7%	Fast	30–60
Lidocaine (Xylocaine)	Amide	2	3.6	7.7	65%	Fast	90–200
Mepivacaine (Carbocaine)	Amide	2	2	7.6	75%	Fast	120–240
Bupivacaine (Marcaine)	Amide	8	30	8.1	95%	Intermediate	180–600
Tetracaine (Pontocaine)	Ester	8	80	8.6	80%	Slow	180–600

*Potency is relative to procaine (1).

Table 3–2 Potential Toxic Effects of Local Anesthetics

- Central nervous system

    Muscle tremors

    Convulsions

    Respiratory depression

    Generalized CNS depression

- Cardiovascular system

    Depression of myocardial contractility

    Hypotension

    Bradycardia

    Ventricular tachycardia/fibrillation: This response has been reported with bupivacaine and may be refractory to treatment and fatal

- Methemoglobinemia

    This response most often is linked to benzocaine but has been reported with other agents

- Allergic reactions

    Associated with para-aminobenzoic acid (PABA), a metabolite of the ester local anesthetics and of methylparaben, a preservative used in many of the local anesthetics

- Tissue toxicity

    Local anesthetic injection has been shown to cause reversible skeletal muscle damage and, rarely, neuronal damage

uncharged base form is most lipid soluble, diffusing readily across the nerve sheath; dissociation is favored by increasing pH. This is why efficacy is decreased in inflamed and infected (low pH) tissues.

Local anesthetic agents show a preferential effect on nerve fibers with the order (most to least sensitive) being preganglionic sympathetic (B fibers) > small sensory (A-delta fibers) > motor (A-alpha fibers). Sensitivity of unmyelinated pain (C) fibers to local anesthetic agents is similar to B fibers, but blockade may be affected by factors other than those influencing the myelinated fibers. Sensation disappears in the order of pain, cold, warmth, touch, then joint and deep pressure and recovers in the reverse order.

Of the many local anesthetic agents available, only a few are commonly used in veterinary medicine, including lidocaine, mepivacaine, and bupivacaine. A topical 5% eutectic mixture of lidocaine and prilocaine (EMLA cream, Astra Pharmaceuticals) applied to unbroken skin also is effective when applied to animals for such procedures as venipuncture but must be applied at least 15–30 min in advance. While many techniques have been described for the common domestic species, Tables 3–3 through 3–5 describe selected local anesthetic techniques that have shown relatively common application for local/regional anesthesia or pain management. Figures 3–1 through 3–4 illustrate the sites for injection for several techniques described in Table 3–3.

Table 3–3   Selected Local Anesthetic Techniques in Dogs and Cats

Nerves	Area Anesthetized	Technique*	Dosage
Infraorbital (Fig. 3–1A)	Upper lip, nose, roof of nasal cavity, skin cranial to infraorbital foramen	Insert needle 1 cm cranial to (and advance to) infraorbital foramen either intra- or extraorally	0.5–2 ml**
Trigeminal (ophthalmic division) (Fig. 3–1C)	Eye, orbit, conjunctiva, eyelids, skin of forehead: glove akinesia may occur	Insert needle ventral to zygomatic process at level of lateral canthus, cranial to ramus of mandible in mediocaudal direction to orbital fissure	1–2 ml**
Maxillary (Fig. 3–1B)	Maxilla, upper teeth and lip, nose	Insert needle at 90° angle ventral to border of zygomatic arch, 0.5 cm caudal to lateral canthus	0.25–1 ml**
Mental (Fig. 3–1E)	Lower lip	Insert needle rostral to mental foramen at level of 2nd premolar	1–2 ml**

Mandibular (inferior alveolar br.) (Fig. 3–1D)	Cheek, canine, incisor teeth, mucosa and skin of chin	Insert needle at lower angle of jaw, 1.5 cm rostral to angular process; advance 1.5 cm dorsally along medial surface of ramus	0.5–1 ml**
Brachial plexus (Fig. 3–2)	Area distal to and including the elbow	22 ga, 7.5 cm needle inserted medial to shoulder joint toward costochondral junction parallel to vertebrae. Inject while withdrawing needle. Aspirate first. Onset requires 20–30 min	4–6 mg/kg (L) 1.5–2 mg/kg (B)
IV regional (BIER-block)	Area distal to tourniquet	Apply tourniquet after desanguination of limb with Esmarch bandage. Inject into superficial vein. Limit to 2 hr	2–3 ml L diluted to 5–10 ml with saline

(continues)

Table 3-3   *(Continued)*

Nerves	Area Anesthetized	Technique*	Dosage
Intercostal	For thoracotomy, rib fractures, pleural space drainage	Block minimum of 5 (2 cranial and 2 caudal to site). Caudal border of rib near intervertebral foramen	0.25–1 ml B per site B: ≤3 mg/kg
Interpleural regional	Same as for intercostal block	Requires placement of interpleural catheter	1–2 ml B
Epidural regional (Fig. 3–3)	Anesthesia caudal to umbilicus	22 ga, 2.5–7.5 cm spinal needle (25 ga hypodermic needle for patients <2 kg). Lumbosacral space: needle introduced on dorsal midline just caudal to line between iliac wings. Needle advanced until distinct "pop" is felt (inter-	1 ml/5 kg L,B; Maximum of 6 ml has been advised

		arcuate ligament). May observe tail flick. Check for CSF (if present decrease dose by 50% or withdraw 1–2 mm)	
Digital block (Fig. 3–4)	Provide analgesia for onychectomy	Superficial radial n: dorsomedial carpus; ulnar n (dorsal cutaneous br): lateral carpus; median n & ulnar n (palmar br): palmar carpus	0.1–0.3 ml B per site ≤3 mg/kg

L = lidocaine; B = bupivacaine

*Use 25 ga needle unless otherwise indicated.

**Dose is for 2% lidocaine or 0.5% bupivacaine in dogs. The dose in cats is 0.25–0.5 ml. Total dosage for lidocaine should not exceed 4–5 mg/kg for lidocaine and 2 mg/kg for bupivacaine for either species.

Table 3-4   Selected Local Anesthetic Techniques in Horses

Nerve(s)	Area Anesthetized	Technique	Dosage*
Supraorbital (frontal)	Upper lid	Insert 25 ga needle into supraorbital foramen located 5–7 cm above medial canthus at depth of 1.5–2 cm, injecting shallow to deep	5 ml
Auriculopalpebral	Akinesia of upper lid only	Insert needle into depression caudal to mandible at ventral edge of zygomatic arch	5 ml
Caudal epidural caudal nn. sacral nn.	Tail, perineum including rectum, vulva, vagina, prevents straining	Insert 18–22 ga hypodermic or spinal needle into 1st intercoccygeal space with needle perpendicular to skin surface or point directed ventrocranial (30°). Placing drop of agent into needle hub will verify proper location as fluid is aspirated into epidural space. Adding xylazine (0.17	0.2–0.3 mg/ kg

mg/kg) or detomidine (0.06 mg/kg) to the lidocaine will increase duration of analgesia

Note: These are just a few commonly used local anesthetic techniques in horses. For descriptions of additional blocks for the head, for diagnostic nerve and joint blocks, and techniques for laparotomy, refer to "Recommended Reading."

*Dosage is for 2% lidocaine.

Table 3–5 Selected Local Anesthetic Techniques in Ruminants and Swine

Nerve(s)	Area Anesthetized	Technique	Dosage*
Infiltration	Paralumbar fossa	Line block of incision site.	50 ml
		Inverted L technique: cranial and dorsal to incision site.	50–100 ml
		Desensitize skin first, then inject deeper to desensitize muscle and peritoneum	
Proximal paravertebral (dorsal and	Paralumbar fossa	Desensitize subcutaneous sites for needle entry with 1–2 ml L. Use 14 ga needle to guide	15 ml deep, 5 ml after withdrawing

(continues)

Table 3-5 *(Continued)*

Nerve(s)	Area Anesthetized	Technique	Dosage*
ventral br. of T13, L1, L2		16–18 ga, 11–15 cm needle. Entry sites are 5 cm off midline (2.5–3 cm for small ruminants). Pass needle down to cranial aspect of transverse process and "walk off" front edge of process (+ 1 cm). T13: front of transverse process of L1 L1: front of transverse process of L2 L2: front of transverse process of L3	needle 1–2 cm, *per site* Small ruminants: 2–3 ml/ site (total dose)
Distal paravertebral (same as for proximal block)	Paralumbar fossa	Nerves are desensitized at distal ends of transverse processes of L1, L2, and L3. 18 ga, 7.5 cm needle is inserted ventral to process and injection made	20 ml ventral, 5 ml dorsal

		in fan-shaped pattern. Needle is withdrawn and reinserted dorsal to process	
IV regional in cattle and small ruminants	Area distal to tourniquet	Apply tourniquet or cuff (>200 mmHg) to limb. Inject into superficial vein with 20–25 ga needle close to surgical site. Apply pressure to site to avoid hematoma. Anesthesia onset is 5–10 min and persists until tourniquet is removed (max: ≤2 hr).	30 ml; 3–10 ml for small ruminants and swine
Peterson eye block abducens, trochlear, oculomotor, ophthalmic, maxillary and mandibular brr. of trigeminal nerve	Eye, orbit, orbicularis oculi muscle. Facilitates enucleation when combined with auriculo-palpebral block	SC infiltration at notch formed by zygomatic and temporal processes of malar bone. Use 14 ga needle inserted at same site as guide for 18 ga, 11 cm needle directed horizontal and slightly posterior to reach solid bone (site of orbitorotundum where nerves exit) and inject	15 ml

(continues)

Table 3-5 *(Continued)*

Nerve(s)	Area Anesthetized	Technique	Dosage*
Auriculolpalpebral	Eyelids	Same site as above. Withdraw needle and redirect posteriorly, lateral to zygomatic arch and inject during insertion to 5–7.5 cm. Upper lid may require local infiltration 2–3 cm from lid margin.	10 ml
Bovine dehorn cornual branch of zygomatico-temporal n. (of trigeminal n.)	Horn and base of horn	Temporal ridge, 2 cm from horn base, depth of 1–2.5 cm. Nerve is palpable here. Inject 2–3 cm rostral to horn with 18 ga needle. Aspirate first. An SC ring block around the horn base may be needed for cosmetic dehorn and large horns	5–10 ml
Caprine dehorn same nerve as previous (1)	Horn and base of horn	1. Halfway between lateral canthus and lateral horn base: insert needle (22	

plus cornual br. of infratrochlear n. (2)		ga, 2.5 cm) close to caudal ridge of supraorbital process 1–1.5 cm deep. 2. Halfway between medial canthus and medial horn base: insert needle dorsal and parallel to dorsomedial margin of orbit, inject in line. Debudding of kids: ring block, 0.5 ml/horn	2–3 ml/site (<10 mg/kg maximum)
Caudal epidural (coccygeal and sacral nn.) ruminants camelids	Tail, perineum including rectum, vulva, vagina, prevents straining	Insert 18–22 ga hypodermic or spinal needle into 1st intercoccygeal space with needle perpendicular to skin surface or point directed ventrocranial (30°). Placing drop of agent into needle hub will verify proper location as fluid is aspirated into epidural space. Adding xylazine (0.05 mg/kg for cattle, 0.17 mg/kg for	5–6 ml: cattle 0.22 mg/kg for llamas and small ruminants

(continues)

Table 3–5 (Continued)

Nerve(s)	Area Anesthetized	Technique	Dosage*
		llamas) to lidocaine will increase duration of analgesia	
Cranial epidural (small ruminants and pigs)	Anesthesia caudal to diaphragm	Technique is similar to that used in dog. Site is between L9 and S1. Onset: 2–15 min. Rear limb paralysis persists up to 2 hr. Reduce dose by 50% if CSF is noted in needle. Requires 18–20 ga, 6–16 cm needle, shortest for small ruminants; longest for large pigs. Swine: xylazine (1–2 mg/kg) or detomidine 0.5 mg/kg) to lidocaine will increase duration of analgesia	2–4 mg/kg (ruminant) 0.8–1 mg/kg (pigs)

SC: subcutaneous
*Dosage is for 2% lidocaine (L).

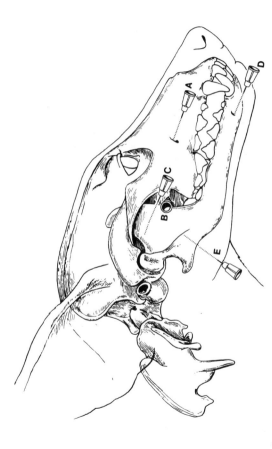

Figure 3–1 Needle placement for local anesthetic injection of the (A) infraorbital, (B) maxillary, (C) ophthamic division of the trigeminal, (D) mental, and (E) mandibular (inferior alveolar branch) nerves. (Reprinted with permission from Thurmon, et al., eds., *Lumb and Jones' Veterinary Anesthesia*, 3rd ed., Baltimore: Williams & Wilkins, 1996, page 430.)

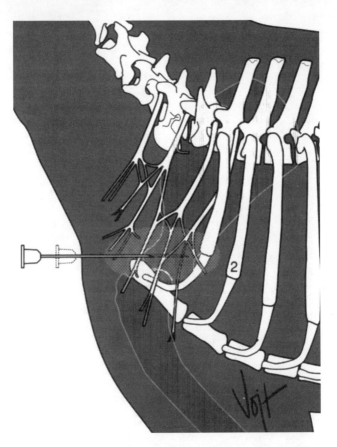

Figure 3-2   Needle placement for brachial plexus block medial to shoulder joint, lateral aspect of left thoracic limb; 2 is the second rib. (Reprinted with permission from Muir and Hubbell, eds., *Handbook of Veterinary Anesthesia*, 2nd ed., St. Louis: Mosby, 1995, page 100.)

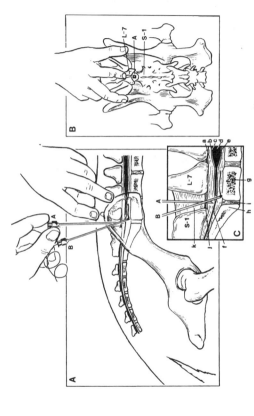

Figure 3–3 Needle placement (A) into the lumbosacral epidural space of dogs and cats. Palpation of the dorsal iliac wings and dorsal process of lumbar vertebra 7 will guide placement on the midline just caudal to a line drawn between the wings and just cranial to the first sacral vertebra. (Reprinted with permission from Thurmon et al., eds., *Lumb and Jones' Veterinary Anesthesia*, 3rd ed., Baltimore: Williams & Wilkins, 1996, page 435.)

Right Forepaw

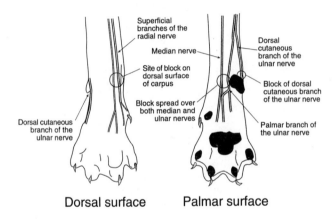

Superficial branches of the radial nerve

Median nerve

Site of block on dorsal surface of carpus

Block spread over both median and ulnar nerves

Dorsal cutaneous branch of the ulnar nerve

Dorsal cutaneous branch of the ulnar nerve

Block of dorsal cutaneous branch of the ulnar nerve

Palmar branch of the ulnar nerve

Dorsal surface

Palmar surface

Figure 3–4 Diagram of right forepaw of a cat illustrating sites for injection of local anesthetic to provide analgesia for onychectomy. (Reprinted with permission from Pascoe, Local and regional anesthesia and analgesia, in *Seminars in Veterinary Medicine and Surgery (Small Animal)* 1997;12(2):435.)

4

Inhalation Agents

Inhalation agents provide the most versatile and readily controlled method of general anesthesia and are especially well suited for prolonged and complex procedures and for common as well as uncommon veterinary species. The anesthetic agents are carried in oxygen; thus, patients receive an enriched oxygen mixture and most often are intubated, which assures a protected airway and provides a method for ventilatory support. The main disadvantages of these agents are the expense of equipment necessary to deliver the agent and, despite the ability to readily control the concentration delivered, vigilant monitoring is essential to avoid excessive anesthetic depth, which can rapidly lead to patient mortality.

Inhalant anesthetics are vapors (a liquid at ambient temperature and pressure; these include all potent inhalant agents) or gases (a gas at ambient temperature and pressure, such as nitrous oxide) administered into the respiratory tract and absorbed from alveoli into the blood to create a partial pressure (tension). *This partial pressure allows the gas to pass from the blood to the brain, where the agents exert reversible generalized central nervous system depression,* the degree of which has been described as depth of anesthesia (Table 4–1).

Some of the physicochemical characteristics determine the action and margin of safety of the agents and dictate how they are supplied and the equipment needed for safe delivery, as well as how they are taken up by the lung, distributed within the body, and eliminated. *Vapor pressure* is a measure of the agent's ability to evaporate (volatility) and must be sufficient to provide adequate concentration in the vapor state to produce anesthesia under ambient conditions. *Saturated vapor pressure* represents the maximum achievable vapor concentration for a given liquid at a given temperature (and barometric pressure); it is determined by dividing vapor pressure by barometric pressure (e.g., Halothane: $244/760 = 32\%$ saturated vapor pressure). The greater is the vapor pressure, the greater the concentration of inhalant deliverable to the patient (and environment).

The *boiling point,* defined as the temperature at which the vapor pressure is equal to atmospheric pressure, is greater than room temperature for all inhalant

Table 4–1 Stages and Characteristics of General Anesthesia

Stage/Description	Pulse Rate	ABP	Respiration	Reflexes Lost	Ocular Reflexes Lost	Muscle Tone
I/Analgesia	⇑	⇑	Regular ±⇑*	All present	All present	Normal
II/Delerium	⇑	⇑	Erratic ±⇑*	All present	Present: nystagmus	Excessive movement
III/Surgical						
Plane 1, light	⇓**	N	⇓	Laryngeal	Diminished	⇓
Planes 2 and 3, medium	⇓⇓**	⇓	⇓	Pedal	Lacrimation, palpebral	⇓⇓
Plane 4, deep	⇓⇓**	⇓⇓	⇓⇓, irregular		Corneal	⇓⇓⇓
IV	⇓⇓⇓	Barely palpable	Apnea			⇓⇓⇓

Note: When unaffected by parenteral agents administered (anticholinergic agents, opioids), pupils are dilated during stages I and II, are normal or constricted in planes 1–3, and are dilated in plane 4 and stage IV. In cattle, eye position is a reliable indicator of depth. The eye moves from central to ventral as surgical anesthetic depth is achieved. As anesthesia becomes deeper, the eye returns to central location.

(continues)

Table 4–1 *(Continued)*

ABP = arterial blood pressure

N = normal

*Breath holding may occur.

**Rate depends on other contributing factors, including premedications, body temperature, fluid balance.

agents except nitrous oxide (N_2O); therefore, all are liquids at room temperature except N_2O, which is supplied for use in blue cylinders compressed to its liquid state at 750 psi. Hence, the pressure gauge on a tank of N_2O does not indicate the quantity of gas remaining until all liquid is converted to a gas state and pressure begins to decrease as the gas empties.

The quantity of inhalant agent delivered is discussed clinically as *concentration in volume percentage,* which represents the percentage of the agent in relation to the carrier gas mixture (oxygen alone or combined with N_2O).

The *molecular weight,* unique for each vapor, is that weight which occupies 22.4 liters under standard conditions (0°C [273 K, absolute scale] and 760 mmHg [barometric pressure at 1 atmosphere sea level]). The *specific gravity* is the ratio of the weight of a unit volume of one substance to a similar volume of water under similar conditions (20°C). Molecular weight and agent specific gravity are properties that allow determination of the volume of vapor yielded by 1 ml of anesthetic liquid (Figure 4–1). From this calculation, the cost of using an inhalant agent may be approximated, based on percentage delivered, total carrier gas flow, and time (see Figure 4–1).

1. 1 ml liquid isoflurane $\times$ 1.49 g/ml (specific gravity) = 1.49 gm

2. 1.49 gm $\div$ 185 (molecular weight) = 0.0081 mol of liquid

3. 0.0081 mol $\times$ 22400 ml/mol (1 mol of gas = 22.4 L) = 181.4 ml at 273 K (0°C)

4. 181.4 ml vapor $\times$ 293/273 K = 194.7 ml vapor/ml liquid isoflurane at 20°C and 760 mmHg

For example, assume 2% isoflurane delivery with total flow (flowmeter setting) of 2 L/minute.

5. 2% $\div$ 100 $\times$ 2 L/minute $\times$ 60 min = 2400 ml isoflurane vapor per hour

6. 2400 ml isoflurane vapor/hr $\div$ 194.7 ml vapor/ml liquid = 12.3 ml liquid/hr

Figure 4–1 Calculations to determine volume of vapor from 1 ml of anesthetic liquid at 20°C (calculations 1–4) and average anesthetic liquid usage per unit time (calculations 5 and 6), using isoflurane as an example.

The *solubility (partition) coefficient*, the extent to which a gas will dissolve in a given solvent, is expressed as a concentration ratio of the anesthetic in the solvent and gas phases. The blood/gas solubility coefficient (Table 4–2) predicts the speed of induction, recovery, and change in anesthetic depth for an inhalant. The lower is the coefficient, the more rapid the action of the agent. The oil/gas solubility coefficient is the ratio of the concentration of an inhalant in oil and gas phases at equilibrium, correlates inversely with anesthetic potency (as represented by the minimum alveolar concentration), and describes the capacity of lipids for the inhalant. The lower is the oil/gas solubility coefficient, the lower the potency and thus the higher the MAC value.

Several factors control anesthetic delivery to the lungs and uptake by the blood; these are summarized in Table 4–3. When equilibrium between delivery and uptake (by blood and tissue) is achieved and the alveolar partial pressure reaches a steady state, the partial pressure in the brain is controlled by the partial pressure in the alveoli.

The *minimum alveolar concentration* (MAC) is a measurement of inhalation agent potency, which refers to the quantity of an agent required to produce a desired effect. MAC, which provides a method for comparing the potency of one agent to another (see Table 4–2), is defined as the minimum alveolar concentration of an anesthetic agent at one atmosphere that produces immobility in 50% of patients exposed to a noxious stimulus.

Table 4–2 Physicochemical Properties and Minimum Alveolar Concentration (MAC) of Inhalant Anesthetic Agents

Property	Desflurane	Enflurane	Halo-thane	Iso-flurane	Metho-xyflurane	Sevo-flurane	N₂O
Molecular weight	168	185	197	185	165	200	44
Liquid specific gravity (20°C; gm/ml)	1.47	1.52	1.86	1.49	1.42	1.52	—
ml vapor/ ml liquid (20°C)	209.7	197.5	227	194.7	206.9	182.7	—
Boiling point (°C)	23.5	57	50	49	105	59	−89
Vapor pressure mmHG at 20°C	664	172	243	240	23	160	—

(continues)

Table 4-2 (Continued)

Property	Desflurane	Enflurane	Halothane	Isoflurane	Methoxyflurane	Sevoflurane	N$_2$O
Blood/gas partition coefficient (37°C)	0.42	2.0	2.54	1.46	15.0	0.68	0.47
Oil/gas partition coefficient (37°C)	18.7	96	224	91	970	47	1.40
MAC* (%)	7.1–9.7	2.0–2.3	0.8–1.1	1.3–1.6	0.23–0.29	2.1–2.6	150–200
Biotransformation (% of metabolites)	0.02	2.4	20–25	0.17	50	3.0	0.004

*MAC varies slightly among species and individuals. The value given is an average or range derived from values reported for several species. As a *general* rule, concentrations required for clinical purposes are approximately 2–3 times the MAC value immediately following induction (mask induction may require 3–5 times MAC) and 1.5–2 times MAC value for anesthetic maintenance.

Table 4–3 Factors That Increase the Rate of Rise of Inhalant Anesthetic Tension (Partial Pressure) in the Alveoli

I. Increased delivery of anesthetic to the lungs

    A. Increased inspired concentration (the higher is the inspired concentration administered, the more rapid the rate of rise of the alveolar concentration)

        1. Increased vaporizer setting

        2. Increased fresh gas inflow (this effect is significant during the induction phase when uptake is significant)

        3. Decreased breathing circuit volume (the smaller is the circuit volume, the more rapidly the inspired concentration is affected by concentration delivered from the vaporizer)

        4. Second gas effect: Passive increase in inspired concentration of an anesthetic gas due to rapid uptake of large volumes of a less soluble agent used in a high concentration (N_2O), therefore the increased concentration accelerates the rate of rise of the second gas in the alveoli; 50% N_2O augments inflow into alveoli and accelerates uptake of the second gas in mixture (e.g., halothane, isoflurane), which is used at much lower concentrations

    B. Increased alveolar ventilation

        1. Occurs with application of mechanical ventilation

        2. Occurs with a decrease in dead space ventilation

        3. Relative to functional residual capacity (FRC; volume remaining in lungs after normal expiration). The smaller is the FRC, the less time it takes to "wash in"

(continues)

Table 4–3   *(Continued)*

the "new" gas mixture. FRC is decreased in pregnancy and in a variety of primary respiratory diseases

II. Decreased removal (uptake) from the alveoli

  A. Decreased blood/gas solubility coefficient

  B. Decreased cardiac output

  C. Decreased alveolar to venous anesthetic partial pressure difference: the magnitude of difference is related to the amount of anesthetic uptake by the tissues and the largest gradient occurs during induction when tissue uptake is greatest

---

Therefore, methoxyflurane (MAC = 0.23) currently is the most potent inhalant agent available. Anesthetic requirements are altered by a variety of factors, which are listed in Table 4–4, but not by duration of anesthesia, sex, or metabolic acid/base or potassium imbalance.

Inhalation agents affect organ systems in addition to the central nervous system. Inhalant agents decrease electrical activity of the cerebral cortex as brain concentration increases, as indicated by decreased frequency and amplitude of EEG activity; however, due to extreme variability, the EEG alone is not a reliable index of anesthetic depth. And, the agent enflurane has epileptogenic potential, which greatly limits its usefulness in veterinary medicine.

Table 4–4   Factors That Affect Anesthetic Requirements (MAC)

Increase in requirements:

Hyperthermia

Hypernatremia

CNS stimulants: amphetamine, ephedrine, physostigmine

Decrease in requirements:

Hypothermia

Hyponatremia

Pregnancy

PaO_2 <40 mmHg

Pa CO_2 >95 mmHg

Mean arterial blood pressure <50 mmHg

Old age

CNS depressants: N_2O, opioids, acepromazine, benzodiazepines, alpha$_2$ agonists, ketamine, thiopental, propofol

---

Inhalants depress *respiratory function* in a dose-dependent manner and respiratory arrest occurs at 2–3 MAC. Of the currently available agents, respiratory depression occurs in the following order from most to least at equipotent concentrations: enflurane > desflurane ≥ isoflurane = methoxyflurane ≥ sevoflurane > halothane. Halothane has been reported to produce a paradoxic tachypnea in some patients, and the mechanism is unknown.

All agents depress *cardiovascular performance* in a dose-dependent manner, associated with a negative inotropic effect, decreased sympathoadrenal activity, and vasodilation. Halothane is noted for its cardiac sensitization to epinephrine-induced arrhythmias. This occurs to a much lesser extent with methoxyflurane and is negligible with the other agents. Vasodilation increases with increasing depth of isoflurane anesthesia, which contributes to hypotension. Myocardial depression is relatively less with isoflurane, desflurane, and sevoflurane than halothane, methoxyflurane, and enflurane. Desflurane, while similar to isoflurane in cardiovascular effects, is reported to sustain autonomic activity better and maintain a relatively constant heart rate and, overall, is most sparing of cardiovascular function.

While all of the inhalation agents are capable of causing *hepatocellular injury* due to reduced oxygen delivery, isoflurane, sevoflurane, and desflurane better maintain hepatic blood flow and oxygenation, especially during prolonged periods. Halothane has been specifically though rarely associated with fulminant hepatic necrosis in humans and some animal species and should be avoided in animals with identified hepatic abnormalities. This effect is probably influenced by such concurrent factors as hypoxemia, N_2O administration, prior induction of hepatic drug-metabolizing enzymes, and mechanical ventilation.

All agents decrease renal blood flow and glomerular filtration rate in a dose-related manner. The effect is exacerbated by preexisting dehydration and hemodynamic abnormalities and may be minimized by intraoperative fluid therapy. Methoxyflurane is most nephrotoxic and was removed from human use for this reason. The cause is associated with methoxyflurane biotransformation, which releases free fluoride ions that cause direct tubular damage resulting in nonoliguric renal failure. Enflurane and sevoflurane also produce free fluoride ions secondary to biotransformation, and sevoflurane yields a nephrotoxic compound, olefin, when it reacts with carbon dioxide absorbents; however, neither seems to result in concentrations great enough to cause significant renal damage.

All potent volatile anesthetic agents can trigger *malignant hyperthermia* but halothane is the most potent of the commonly used agents. Malignant hyperthermia is a pharmacogenetic, often fatal, myopathy of humans and swine typically characterized by increased temperature, muscle rigidity, metabolic acidosis, hyperkalemia, and striated muscle deterioration due to a defect in calcium homeostasis at the cellular level. It has been reported in horses, dogs, cats, birds, deer, and other wildlife species, but a genetic link has not been elucidated in these species. In wildlife species, the syndrome is referred to as *capture myopathy*.

Anesthetic elimination (and recovery) is influenced by alveolar ventilation, cardiac output, agent solubility, and duration of anesthesia (the longer is the duration, the greater the extent of tissue saturation). When a rebreathing circuit is used (Chapter 5), purging the circuit with oxygen by engaging the oxygen flush valve or increasing oxygen flow rate will facilitate elimination as will continued assisted ventilation. While it may seem intuitive to simply disconnect the patient from the breathing system, this deprives the patient of oxygen supplementation and increases contamination of the work environment with exhaled anesthetic agent.

Biotransformation is unique to each anesthetic agent (see Table 4–2) and occurs primarily in the liver. The potential for acute and chronic toxicities (Table 4–5) associated with environmental exposure to inhaled agents increases with increased biotransformation to metabolites. This is a major reason why methoxyflurane (metabolized up to 50%) no longer is used in human

Table 4–5   Adverse Side Effects Associated with Environmental Exposure to Inhalation Agents

Reproduction disorders	Abortion, malformations
Malignancy	
Vital organ dysfunction	Hepatopathy, renal pathologic changes, behavioral changes (headache, fatigue, decreased performance)
N_2O	Neutropenia, megaloblastic anemia (decreased vitamin B_{12} & methionine synthetase synthesis

medicine and has lost favor in veterinary medicine, representing a significant health hazard to patients and personnel. Practices to minimize workplace contamination (Table 4–6) with inhalant agents should be utilized to minimize human exposure.

Table 4–6   Work Practices That Help Minimize Environmental Contamination of the Workplace with Inhalant Anesthetics

1. Use a scavenger system
2. Educate all personnel about the potential health hazards
3. Keep equipment and vaporizers in good condition
4. Identify and repair leaks in system by an established routine
5. Fill vaporizers at the end of the day
6. Fill vaporizers in a well-ventilated area
7. Inflate endotracheal tube cuffs adequately
8. Avoid the use of mask and chamber inductions and maintenance whenever possible
9. Keep patients on O_2 as long as possible to scavenge expired anesthetic gases
10. Avoid or minimize exposure with the use of respirators with organic vapor cartridges (available from medical supply companies) during the first trimester of pregnancy (while the first trimester is the most vulnerable period, steps to minimize exposure should be practiced throughout the pregnancy)

Nitrous oxide will not provide general anesthesia alone due to its low potency (see Table 4–2) but is used as a percentage of the carrier gas (50–70%) to decrease requirements of the more potent agents and speed induction, due to its second gas effect (see Table 4–3). While cardiopulmonary effects are minimal, some contraindications are associated with its use and it has been associated with specific toxic effects (see Table 4–5). Nitrous oxide rapidly diffuses into closed gas spaces (while nitrogen slowly diffuses out) and will cause expansion of the space and respiratory compromise (e.g., pneumothorax, intestinal obstruction); therefore, it is contraindicated in these situations. Nitrous oxide rarely is used in large animal species because of the large volume of gas contained in the gastrointestinal tract and potential for excessive distension as well as the need for 100% oxygen to maintain adequate oxygenation during inhalation anesthesia. Diffusion hypoxia can occur with N_2O use, due to its rapid exit from the blood into the lungs when delivery is ended. It is essential that 100% oxygen delivery be continued for *at least 5 min* after N_2O is discontinued.

Inhalant agents offer the most versatile method for maintenance of anesthesia available today. Isoflurane currently is the most commonly used and favored agent in veterinary medicine, although sevoflurane, with its lower solubility, offers benefits that may rival isoflurane when it becomes a more economical option. Halothane remains in common use, despite its arrhythmogenic potential, slower onset and cessation of action, and greater potential for cardiovascular depression. Halothane historically has been preferred in equine anesthesia, at least for elective procedures, due to reports of smoother recoveries (than isoflurane). Recently, use of sevoflurane has been reported to produce smooth, rapid recoveries and may gain widespread use in equine anesthesia in the future. Inhalant anesthesia requires vigilant monitoring (Chapter 6) and is not without potential detrimental effects to both the patient and the work environment.

5

Anesthetic Equipment

The Anesthesia Machine

Basic components of an anesthesia machine include a compressed gas source, pressure-reducing valve (pressure regulator), flowmeter, and vaporizer. Compressed (carrier, fresh) gas sources are oxygen and N_2O. While N_2O commonly is used in human anesthesia, use in veterinary medicine is limited mainly to dogs and cats to spare requirements for the more potent inhalant agents. In addition to liquid bulk tanks for oxygen, sources include *large tanks* (e.g., H tanks with 6,910 L capacity for oxygen or 14,520 L for N_2O) connected by high-pressure, color-coded (green for oxygen, blue for N_2O) hose known as DISS (diameter index and safety system) and *small tanks* (E tanks: 655 L capacity for oxygen, 1,590 L for N_2O), which may be connected, via a hanger yolk with a self-contained pressure regulator and pressure gauge, directly to a small animal machine. A pin index system configuration (Figure 5–1) prevents inadvertent interchange of medical gases. Compressed gas tanks are filled under pressure (2200 psi for oxygen; 750 psi for N_2O) and always must be handled carefully. The pressure gauge reading for oxygen tanks decreases linearly with decreasing content, providing an indication of available oxygen remaining.

Pressure regulators reduce the pressure exiting the compressed gas source to a constant and safe pressure of 50–60 psi to provide a constant pressure to the flowmeter. *Flowmeters* control and indicate the rate of flow of oxygen and N_2O delivered to the common gas outlet or through an out-of-system vaporizer. Gas moves from bottom to top around a float, which indicates flow rate in L (or ml)/min. Most flowmeter floats are cylindrical and read in the middle; alternate-shaped floats are read at the top. Flowmeters are calibrated at 20°C and 760 mmHg. Flow knobs usually are color coded and oxygen flowmeter knobs usually are larger than other knobs on the machine to minimize human error.

Vaporizers deliver a controlled concentration of potent inhalant to the patient breathing system. Currently, the safest vaporizers are out of (breathing) circle (VOC; Figure 5–2), precision, agent specific, concentration

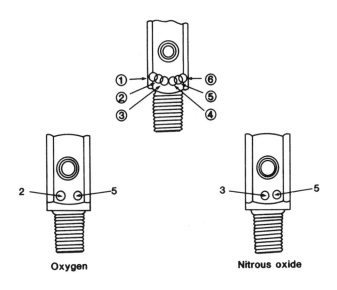

Figure 5–1 Diagram of the pin index safety system, illustrating the spacing between the valve outlet and pin holes in the valve bodies for oxygen and N$_2$O cylinders. The numbering system identifies each pin hole site. (Reprinted with permission from CE Short, *Principles and Practice of Veterinary Anesthesia*, Baltimore: Williams & Wilkins, 1987, page 397.)

calibrated, and variable bypass, which are temperature, flow, and back-pressure compensated. Because vaporizers different than those just described remain in use in veterinary practice, we provide a brief review of these vaporizers.

The two major exceptions that remain in veterinary medical use are nonprecision in-the-circle vaporizers (Stephens, Ohio #8) and multiagent measured-flow, out-of-circle vaporizers (Copper Kettle, Vernitrol). In-the-circle vaporizers (VIC) almost always are located on the inspiratory side of the breathing system and the patient breathes through the vaporizer. Vaporization and anesthetic concentration in the breathing system is controlled by patient ventilation (increased ventilation will increase vaporization); the arbitrary settings on the vaporizers (Ohio #8, 0–10; Stephens, off–8) indicate the amount of inspiratory flow diverted into the vaporization chamber. These vaporizers are nonprecision, low resistance, and not temperature compensated, meaning the delivered concentration is unknown and can change unpredictably, the anesthesia often being referred to as *qualitative* (versus quantitative). Inspired concentration *increases* with increased temperature, increased ventilation (spontaneous or mechanical), and decreased fresh gas flow into the breathing circuit. Mechanical ventilation is contraindicated with VICs. The Ohio #8, with its wick to increase surface area, was designed specifically for methoxyflurane (low volatility). Guidelines for use

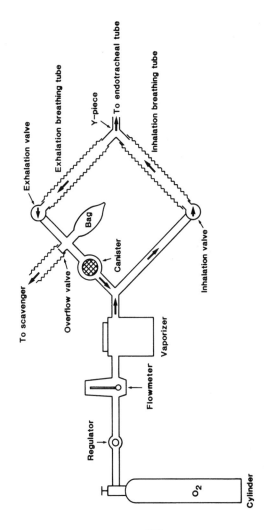

Figure 5–2 Diagram of vaporizer and breathing component location for VOC (vaporizer out of circle). (Reprinted with permission from CE Short, *Principles and Practice of Veterinary Anesthesia*, Baltimore: Williams & Wilkins, 1987, page 403.)

with isoflurane and halothane (*with wick removed*) have been published; however, this practice is discouraged due to the high volatility of these agents and the increased potential to deliver fatal concentrations. The Stephens vaporizer has been used for halothane and isoflurane (and sevoflurane) and is intended for use with a low-flow circle breathing system. A wick is provided for use with methoxyflurane as well. Vigilant monitoring will help assure that excessive concentrations are not delivered to the patient.

Measured-flow vaporizers allow use of multiple agents because they contain two oxygen flowmeters, one for diluent flow and one for vaporizer flow. The appropriate flow setting for both flowmeters must be calculated to deliver the desired concentration of the specific agent used (Figure 5–3). Originally, a special circular slide rule to determine flowmeter settings was included with these vaporizers (see Figure 5–3).

Two other features of anesthesia machines need mention. While not essential, most anesthesia machines have an *oxygen flush valve* (OFV), which supplies oxygen to the common gas outlet or directly to the breathing circuit at an unmetered rate of 35–75 L/min. The OFV flow bypasses the vaporizer in contemporary machines, but older machines to which precision vaporizers were added later may direct oxygen, with flush activation, through the vaporizer, with the potential to increase anesthetic output if the vaporizer is turned on. When using an anesthesia machine, the circuitry should be

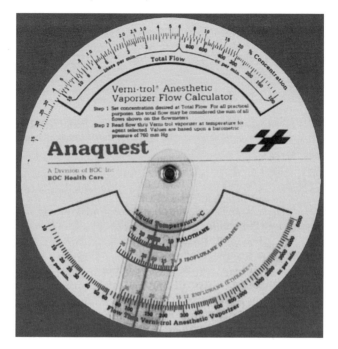

Figure 5–3 Circular slide rule for calculation of oxygen flows for an anesthetic machine with a measured-flow VOC vaporizer (Verni-trol, Copper Kettle). The rule can be used for multiple anesthetic agents and a variety of total oxygen flow rates over a range of temperatures. Calculations can be made according to the following equations (using halothane as the anesthetic agent):

1. Saturated vapor pressure (halothane) = 243 ÷ 760 = 32%; desired TGF (total gas flow) = 2 L/min; desired halothane concentration [%Hal] = 1.5%

2. Halothane vapor leaving vaporizer = desired %Hal × TGF = 1.5% × 2000 ml = 30 ml

(continues)

Figure 5–3 *(Continued)*

3. To provide 30 ml halothane vapor leaving vaporizer: TGF exiting vaporizer = 30 ml ÷ 32%(sat VP) = 94 ml.

4. 94 ml (TGF exiting vaporizer) − 30 ml (halothane vapor) = *64 ml oxygen entering vaporization chamber (vaporizer flowmeter setting).*

5. *Bypass oxygen flowmeter setting* = 2000 ml (total flow) − 94 ml = *1906 ml*

(Reprinted with permission from Thurmon et al., eds., *Lumb and Jones' Veterinary Anesthesia,* 3rd ed., Baltimore: Williams and Wilkins, 1996, page 387.)

followed and understood prior to use. The OFV is used to flush (remove) anesthetic from the rebreathing system during recovery or when problems with anesthetic depth are identified; using it to fill the rebreathing bag in an attempt to ventilate and deepen the patient's anesthesia is ineffective, as its purpose is to dilute anesthetic concentration within the breathing circle. The OFV should not be used in pediatric circuits or nonrebreathing systems, both of which have small volumes, due to the danger of overpressurizing the patient's respiratory system. The *common gas outlet* is the site from which gases that have passed through the flowmeter, vaporizer (VOC), or OFV exit the anesthesia machine for delivery to the breathing system. Some vaporizers, purchased separately and added to a machine, have been placed between the common gas outlet and the breathing circuit, which increases the risk of delivering excessive concentrations should the vaporizer be tilted or the oxygen flush valve engaged when the vaporizer is on.

Anesthesia Breathing Systems

The breathing system connects the anesthesia machine (via the fresh gas inlet) to the patient (via mask or endotracheal tube). Two types of circuits are used in veterinary medicine. The *circle rebreathing system* is the most common circuit used and is standard equipment on most anesthesia machines. Pediatric, standard adult (small animal), and large animal circuits differ primarily in their internal diameters, rebreathing bag, and overall volume and size of the carbon dioxide absorbent canister. Pediatric and adult circuits have the same size absorbent canister and differ only in the size of the breathing tubes and rebreathing bag used (Table 5–1).

Circle systems have the same basic components, including:

- The Y-piece (patient connection).
- Two breathing tubes (between the Y-piece and one-way valves).
- Paired one-way valves (inspiratory and expiratory), which prevent rebreathing of exhaled gases before they pass through the absorbent canister.
- Fresh gas inlet (site of entry of gases from the common gas outlet).

Table 5-1 Sizes and Recommendations for Fresh Gas Flow Rates of Circle Systems and Nonrebreathing Systems

System	Breathing Diameter Tube	Rebreathing Bag Volume*	Patient Size	Fresh Gas Flow Rate (ml/kg/min)
Circle				
Pediatric	15 mm	0.5–1 L	<7kg	4–11 (closed)
Adult	22 mm	1 L	8–15 kg	10–20 (low flow)
		2 L	16–30 kg	25–35 (semi-closed)
		3 L	31–45 kg	
		5 L	46–135 kg	
		15 and 20 L	135–330 kg	6–10
Large animal	50 mm	30 L	>330	
			<5–7 kg	200–600**
Nonrebreathing				
Bains system (Mapleson classification Type D, modified) Ayre's T-piece (Mapleson classification Type E) Norman elbow				

(Mapleson classification
Type E) Jackson-Rees
System (a modified
Ayre's T-piece; Mapleson
classification Type E)

*Rebreathing bag size may be estimated by multiplying 6 × tidal volume (10 ml/kg) × BW (kg).

**Recommendations for total fresh gas flow are quite variable in the literature but, in general, are 2–3 times minute ventilation (170–350 ml/kg/minute for dogs and cats) to prevent rebreathing of carbon dioxide.

- Pop-off (relief) valve, which vents gases to the scavenger system and prevents excessive pressure within the system.

- Rebreathing bag, which provides peak demands during inspiration, a mechanism for manually assisting ventilation, and a method for observing spontaneous ventilation.

- Pressure manometer, usually attached at absorbent canister and calibrated in cm H_2O to assess pressure achieved during assisted ventilation.

- Absorbent canister.

The absorbent canister is filled with either soda lime or barium lime granules (calcium hydroxide is the primary component of both), which neutralize exhaled CO_2. The reaction ($CO_2 + H_2O \rightarrow H_2CO_3 + 2NaOH + Ca(OH)2 \rightarrow CaCO_2 + Na_2CO_3 + 4H_2O +$ heat) is exhaustive and produces a change in the granules, including heat generation, soft to hard, and a color change (most often white to violet). As a general rule, absorbent granules should be changed after 6–8 hr of use or when the color reaction is apparent in approximately two thirds of the granules.

Nonrebreathing systems have no chemical absorbent and depend on a high fresh-gas flow rate to remove exhaled CO_2 from the breathing system. They are less efficient than the rebreathing system; the oxygen and anesthetic agent are wasted; more anesthetic agent must be scavenged, with a greater potential for environmental contamination; and patient heat and humidity is not conserved, so that patient cooling due to convective heat loss is greater. *The main advantage is less resistance to breathing*; hence, the recommendation for use in small (<5–7 kg) patients. They also are lightweight, easy to position, inexpensive (to purchase), and allow rapid changes in inspired anesthetic concentration. Several systems, classified collectively by the Mapleson system, are available; in general, only four are used in veterinary medicine (see Table 5–1), with the Bains coaxial system being the most popular. The Bains system is a tube (inspired fresh gas delivery) within a tube (carries exhaled gases away from the patient to the reservoir bag and scavenging system) and can be fitted with a pressure manometer (with an additional equipment piece that also has a relief valve and accommodates the reservoir bag).

Waste Gas Scavenging

Several medical problems have been linked to exposure to waste anesthetic gases (see Table 4–5). Guidelines to minimize workplace contamination (see Table 4–6) include a scavenging system on all anesthesia machines to collect and eliminate waste gases from the workplace. A gas-collecting connection (the pop-off or relief valve), an interface, and a disposal system compose the scavenging system assembly. The interface prevents transfer of pressure changes from the disposal system to the breathing system. It includes positive and negative pressure relief mechanisms and, for active systems, a reservoir bag to provide visual assessment of its proper function.

Disposal systems are passive or active. Passive systems include piping waste gases into nonrecirculating ventilation systems, directly to the atmosphere, and through absorption devices (F/air canisters are portable and neutralize inhaled gases with the exception of N_2O but have a limited useful life, making them expensive and variable in effectiveness).

Active systems include piped vacuum and active duct systems. A piped vacuum system is convenient when already in place and when location of exit for passive discharge is inconvenient. An active duct system with high volume flow and low negative pressure is ideal for waste gas removal. Tubing for the connecting parts of the scavenging system ideally should be readily discernible from the breathing circuit. Table 5–2 is a simple guide to performing routine checks of the anesthesia machine and to detecting leaks from the breathing circuit.

Ventilators

Controlled ventilation is unnecessary for the majority of anesthetized veterinary patients, but a variety of patient circumstances will prompt the need for intermittent positive pressure ventilation (IPPV). Indications include apnea; documentation of severe hypoventilation ($\uparrow PaCO_2$); intrathoracic surgery; patient factors such as

Table 5–2 Recommendations for Routine Assessment of Anesthesia Machine and Breathing Circuit to Minimize Risk of Malfunction and Environmental Pollution

1. Machine check
   a. Check anesthetic level in vaporizer and fill if indicated (preferably, at time when room is not in use).
   b. Check tightness of filler cap.
   c. Make sure vaporizer setting is in off position.
2. Oxygen supply and delivery
   a. Check cylinder pressure (50–60 psi) and assess quantity of oxygen available.
   b. For machines equipped with N_2O source and flowmeter, turn on N_2O flow and turn off oxygen supply; N_2O float should drop to zero. (This should be performed at least weekly.)
   c. Verify proper flowmeter function. Float should move freely the entire length of flowmeter tube.
3. Check breathing circuit
   a. Assure all fittings are tight.
   b. Check absorbant canister for need to change soda lime and assure canister is properly positioned and tightly fitted.
   c. Confirm proper function of unidirectional valves of circle by inhaling and exhaling through Y-piece and observing appropriate movement.
   d. Check for leaks: Close the relief valve, occlude the Y-piece, pressurize the circuit to 30 cm H_2O; pressure should remain stable or drop slowly (<250 ml/min). Open the relief valve to assure release of pressure.

(continues)

Table 5–2   *(Continued)*

4. Check waste gas scavenging system
   a. Confirm connection to relief valve.
   b. Connect or activate active scavenging system or verify patency of passive system.
5. Check ventilator function (when applicable).
   a. Turn on prior to connection to breathing circuit (may require partially occluding connecting tubing) to assure function and appropriate settings.
   b. Verify proper connection to breathing circuit, which includes closing the relief valve.
   c. The scavenging system must be connected to the ventilator relief valve when in use.

obesity, abdominal distention, or primary lung dysfunction; use of an intraoperative neuromuscular blocking agent; surgery lasting more than 90 min; the need for hyperventilation in cases of head trauma; and facilitation of a stable plane of surgical anesthesia by enhancing anesthetic agent delivery and uptake.

Maintaining a $PaCO_2$ between 35 and 45 mmHg is the general goal of IPPV; however, there is controversy regarding the desired high-end range for $PaCO_2$, with 50 mmHg commonly recommended. Moderate increases in $PaCO_2$ support arterial blood pressure through endogenous catecholamine release. Intermittent positive pressure ventilation decreases cardiovascular function by impeding venous return to the heart (and therefore diastolic filling). The benefits of IPPV, compared to the potential detrimental effects, should be considered in every patient. High-risk patients with inadequate vascular volume or compromised cardiac function may not tolerate IPPV well, as evidenced by exacerbation of low arterial blood pressure values.

Even though IPPV has a negative effect on cardiovascular performance, this is minimized by assuring adequate intravascular volume, using inotropes to enhance cardiovascular performance (Chapter 7), and applying IPPV within the recommended guidelines (Table 5–3).

Ventilators are classified broadly, based on mode of operation, including pressure cycled and volume cycled. Ventilators require electricity, compressed gas, or both for operation. The timing of *pressure-cycled ventilators* is influenced by a preset peak inspiratory pressure limit. Inspiration will continue until a preset pressure is achieved, regardless of the volume delivered. While this type of operation is safer, in that it will not allow delivery of excessive pressure during the inspiratory phase, tidal volume delivered may be inadequate (depending on lung and breathing system compliance). The tidal volume delivered tends to decrease over time unless the ventilator periodically is reset to compensate for the temporal decrease in lung compliance.

Volume-cycled ventilators deliver a preset tidal volume regardless of peak pressure achieved. Most ventilators of

Table 5–3 Recommended Settings for Mechanical Ventilation

Setting	Guidelines
Tidal volume*	15–20 ml/kg (small animals)
	10–15 ml/kg (large animals)
Inspiratory time	<1.5 sec (small animals)
	<3 sec (large animals)
I:E (inspiratory to expiratory) ratio	≤1:2
Peak inspiratory pressure	12–20 cm H_2O (small animals)
	20–30 cm H_2O (large animals)
Respiratory frequency	8–14 (dogs)
	10–14 (cats)
	6–10 (horse and cow)
	8–12 (small ruminants and pigs)

*Ventilator tidal volume is set slightly higher than the actual patient needs, to allow for increases in breathing system and airway volume when positive pressure is delivered. Setting tidal volume too low will permit development of atelectasis. When lower tidal volume must be used (e.g., on animals with abdominal distention or diaphragmatic hernia), the rate should be increased accordingly.

this type have settings that limit the maximum pressure achieved to assure patient safety. Maximum pressure during the inspiratory phase increases as patient compliance decreases. Leaks in the breathing circuit do not become readily apparent with volume-cycled operation, while leaks usually are readily apparent with pressure-cycled ventilators.

While ventilators historically have been classified as pressure or volume cycled, the terms are somewhat misleading because most often a timing mechanism controls the change from the inspiratory phase to the expiratory phase, with inspiratory time being a major determinant of the cycle. Ventilators also are classified according to *direction of bellows movement during expiration.* Ascending (during expiration) bellows are considered safer, because they will not fill if a disconnection occurs in the breathing circuit, thus quickly alerting the anesthetist to a problem.

Even though an anesthetized animal may appear to be ventilating adequately, as indicated by a normal spontaneous respiratory rate and a "normal"-appearing tidal volume, some degree of respiratory depression is present. The subsequent elevation of $PaCO_2$ may be quantitated by arterial blood gas analysis or continuously reading capnometers, which visually display a value for end-tidal carbon dioxide, an indirect measure of $PaCO_2$. Anesthesia-associated hypercapnia during spontaneous ventilation tends to increase with the duration of the anesthesia. This stresses the importance of minimizing anesthesia time and providing ventilatory support, either manually or mechanically, for prolonged procedures and high-risk patients.

6

Monitoring Anesthesia

Based on suggestions by the American College of Veterinary Anesthesiologists (ACVA) for monitoring anesthetized veterinary patients, personnel should be "aware of the patient's status at all times during anesthesia and recovery." No monitoring tool or device can take the place of constant human observation; available equipment is meant to enhance the observation skills of the attending anesthetist. Keeping a record of perianesthetic events (see Figure 1–1) will provide a legal document and facilitate appropriate observation and temporal recording of relevant measured parameters and events. Monitoring provides ongoing determination of patient physiologic status, allowing early recognition and treatment of abnormalities and a way to assess therapeutic efficacy. Recommended monitoring methods and devices are targeted to assure adequate circulation, oxygenation, and ventilation. The best treatment for anesthetic complications is prevention. But, when they do occur, early recognition usually will allow correction with minimal intervention and long-term detrimental effects.

Monitoring efforts concentrate on three body systems—the central nervous system (including ocular, musculoskeletal, and other reflexes), the cardiovascular system, and the respiratory system—and should include periodic temperature assessment. The following guidelines should be considered:

1. Evaluation of integrated responses, using one or more parameters for multiple body system assessment, allows more accurate and representative ongoing patient assessment than reliance on a single parameter.

2. Even though a variety of monitoring devices is available, it is best to choose one or two for routine use and become familiar with their benefits and limitations, remembering that they are a supplement to monitoring *not* a replacement.

3. The monitoring plan should increase in complexity (more quantitative measurements) as patient and procedure risk increase.

4. Noninvasive monitors are relatively easy to use but results can be highly variable; the data provided are

best viewed as trends (qualitative) over time rather than quantitative measurements.

5. In general, invasive monitoring techniques are more accurate but more expensive to provide, require greater technical skill, and usually are reserved for high-risk patients and procedures (horses are an exception, for which invasive arterial blood pressure monitoring is used routinely during inhalation anesthesia regardless of patient status).

6. Keeping an anesthetic record provides a method of tracking trends in measured parameters (e.g., heart rate, respiratory rate, blood pressure) and provides information for subsequent anesthetic episodes in that patient.

Signs of the various stages of inhalation anesthesia are listed in Table 4–1. *General anesthesia includes unconsciousness, insensitivity to pain, muscle relaxation, and absence of reflex response.* The degree required for each of these effects depends largely on the procedure. While no clear line divides stages and planes of anesthesia, planes 2 and 3 of stage III are the desired levels for most procedures. Confounding factors that complicate evaluation according to stage, include variation in species response to anesthetic agents, premedication agents administered, PaO_2 and $PaCO_2$ values, and the patient's physical status.

Table 6–1 Parameters Monitored and Applicable Techniques Used During General Anesthesia

Parameter	Method	Comments
Respiratory monitoring		
Respiratory rate, depth, and character	Thoracic movement	Subjective only. No indication of adequacy of ventilation.
	Rebreathing bag movement	Appropriate for assessing changes over time.
	Esophageal stethoscope	May be attached to earpieces or amplifier; also detects heart sounds
	Respiratory (apnea) monitor	Interfaced between ET tube and breathing system. Detects exhaled breath by change in temperature and provides an audible beep. May not be sensitive enough for very small patients.
Tidal and minute volume	Ventilometry	Ventilometer is applied to expiratory side of patient breathing circuit
End-tidal CO_2 (ETCO$_2$)	Capnometry	Provides breathing rate and ETCO$_2$ value.

Hemoglobin saturation (SaO_2 or SpO_2)	Capnography	Also displays graph of expired CO_2 (Figure 6–1)
	Pulse oximeter	Hemoglobin oxygen saturation and pulse rate
Arterial blood gas analysis ($PaCO_2$ and PaO_2)	Laboratory blood gas analyzer	Most accurate assessment of adequacy of ventilation and blood oxygenation
	Handheld analyzers	
Cardiovascular monitoring		
Heart rate	Precordial auscultation	
	Esophageal stethoscope	
	ECG	Also available with self-contained ECG leads (*Heska Corp, Fort Collins, CO*)
		Records myocardial electrical activity but gives no indication of adequacy of perfusion
Pulse rate and quality	Palpation	Subjective; sites vary among species:
		Canine—dorsal pedal, lingual, femoral
		Feline—femoral, ± lingual and dorsal pedal

(continues)

Table 6–1 *(Continued)*

Parameter	Method	Comments
	Pulse oximetry	Equine—facial, transverse facial, dorsal metatarsal Ruminant—auricular, coccygeal, digital Swine—femoral, auricular, coccygeal, brachial Provides pulse rate and indirect assessment of blood oxygenation (SaO_2; Figure 6–2)
Arterial blood pressure (ABP)	Noninvasive	Two methods (both require cuff*): 1. Oscillometric—provides heart rate plus systolic, mean, and diastolic ABP at preset intervals. 2. Doppler crystal probe—applied over artery distal to a cuff with manometer. Skin over artery must be closely clipped, gel applied and probe taped in place, which amplifies sound of pulse. Reliably

measures systolic ABP only.** Also provides continuous auditory information on pulse rhythm and quality. Less automated than oscillometric technique.

Provides continuous, accurate readout of SAP, MAP, and DAP. Requires arterial catheter attached to a pressure transducer and recording device or sphygmomanometer (MAP only) via saline-filled tubing. Sensitive monitor of anesthetic depth, especially useful in horses.

Sites for arterial catheterization:
Canine—dorsal pedal, lingual, femoral
Feline—femoral, dorsal pedal
Equine—facial, transverse facial, dorsal metatarsal

(continues)

Invasive†

Table 6–1 (Continued)

Parameter	Method	Comments
Central venous pressure (CVP)	Measured with catheter placed into anterior vena cava via jugular vein and connected to manometer or pressure transducer zeroed at thoracic inlet	Ruminant–auricular Swine–auricular, femoral Reflects the balance between blood volume and capacity and helps avoid pulmonary edema and overhydration with rapid fluid administration in high-risk patients. *Normal values:* 0–10 cm H_2O (small animal) 5–15 cm H_2O (awake horses) 25–35 cm H_2O (anesthetized horses)
Urine output	Urinary catheter connected to closed collection system	Indirect measure of organ perfusion. Especially important in renal disease. *Normal:* 1–2 ml/kg/hr

Notes: The goal of respiratory monitoring is to determine and maintain adequacy of ventilation (normal $PaCO_2$ and PaO_2). The goal of cardiovascular monitoring is to monitor the electrical activity of the heart and ensure adequate perfusion of vital organs, particularly the brain, heart, and kidneys.

SAP = systolic ABP; MAP = mean ABP; DAP = diastolic ABP.

*Cuff width is approximately 40% the circumference of the appendage.

**As a general rule, when the systolic ABP is 90–100 mmHg, mean ABP is 60–70 mmHg.

†A minimum mean ABP of 60–70 mmHg is considered necessary to assure perfusion of vital organs in *all* species. Cattle may demonstrate higher values during general anesthesia and recumbency, especially as duration of anesthesia increases (e.g., mean ABP = 100–150 mmHg). Horses have been reported to exhibit high values, which increase over time in association with tourniquet application (starting approximately 45 min after tourniquet placement).

Assessment of the cardiovascular and respiratory systems incorporate subjective and objective data that indicate the state of circulation, oxygenation, and ventilation. Table 6–1 lists the parameters that may be assessed and methods and equipment available. Table 6–2 provides details on the principles and operation of the capnograph and pulse oximeter. Table 6–3 lists normal values for some measured parameters in a variety of species. Table 6–4 lists some potential abnormalities that may develop during general anesthesia, potential causes to be investigated, and an approach to management.

Table 6–2   Principles of Operation and Significance of Information Provided by Monitoring Equipment Used in Veterinary Medicine

Equipment	Principles of Operation	Probe Site(s)/Source of Error
Capnography (Figure 6–1)	Infrared absorption is the most common measuring method to determine CO_2 in expired gases. $ETCO_2$ represents alveolar CO_2, which equilibrates with $PaCO_2$, reflecting ventilatory efficiency. Normal capnogram requires metabolism, circulation, and ventilation and it thus monitors multiple vital functions.	Two analyzer types placed between ET tube and breathing circuit: 1. Sidestream—aspirates gases into analyzer via tubing (50–250 ml/min), resulting in lag time. 2. Mainstream—measures CO_2 directly in airway, no lag time. *Error:* $ETCO_2$ underestimates $PaCO_2$ by approximately 5 mmHg (up to 14 in horses) due to alveolar dead space. Ideally, it is a good idea to assess actual $PaCO_2$ periodically during use.
Pulse oximetry (SaO_2 or SpO_2) (Figure 6–2)	Estimates oxygenated hemoglobin (Hgb) as a percent of total hemoglobin. Based on principle that oxygenated and	Two probe types: 1. Transmittance—sends and receives light across tissue: tongue, toe web, ear, vulva.

(continues)

Table 6–2 (Continued)

Equipment	Principles of Operation	Probe Site(s)/Source of Error
	deoxygenated Hgb absorb light differently at different wavelengths, 660 nm (red) and 940 nm (infrared). Requires pulsatile blood. Hemoglobin saturation reflects blood oxygenation (PaO$_2$) as represented by the oxyhemoglobin dissociation curve (Figure 6–2).	2. Reflectance—sends and receives light on the same plane: esophagus, rectum, mucous membranes. *Error:* 1. Low pulse pressure. 2. Increased venous pulsations (e.g., right-heart failure, tourniquet). 3. Cardiac arrhythmias. 4. Movement. 5. Dyshemoglobins (e.g., methemoglobin, carboxyhemoglobin). 6. Dyes (e.g., methylene blue). 7. Anemia (<5 gm/dl). 8. External light. 9. Electrocautery units. 10. Poor probe positioning

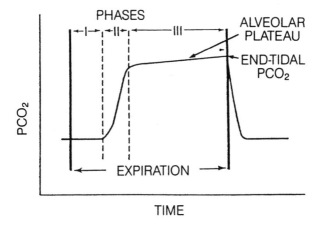

Figure 6–1 Diagram of normal expired CO_2 waveform. The three phases of the normal waveform include apparatus and anatomical series dead space (phase I), mixture of anatomical series and alveolar parallel gas (phase II), and the alveolar plateau (phase III), a mixture of gases from well-perfused alveoli and alveolar dead space (unperfused alveoli). (Reprinted with permission from KK Tremper, Interpretation of noninvasive oxygen and carbon dioxide data. *Can J Anaesth* 1990;37(4):Slxxxi.)

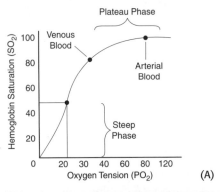

(A)

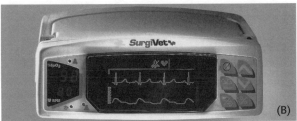

(B)

Figure 6–2 (A) The oxyhemoglobin dissociation curve illustrates the relationship between blood oxygen tension (PO_2) and hemoglobin saturation (SaO_2). A simple guide summarizing the relationship between PaO_2 and SaO_2 follows for interpretation of pulse oximeter readings obtained during clinical monitoring.

PaO₂ (mmHg)	SaO₂ (%)	Interpretation
>80	>95	Normal
<60	<90	Significant hypoxemia
<40	<75	Serious life-threatening hypoxemia

(B) A combination pulse oximeter and electrocardiograph. (Courtesy of SurgiVet Inc., Waukesha, WI.)

Table 6–3 "Normal" Values for Selected Measured Parameters in a Variety of Species

Parameter	Dog	Cat	Horse	Cow	Goat/Sheep	Pig	Rabbit
Temperature (core °C)	37–40	37–40	37–38	37–39	37–40	38–40	38–40
Heart rate/min*	70–140	100–200	25–50	60–80	60–90	60–90	200–325
Respiratory rate/min	10–30	12–40	8–15	12–30	15–30	10–30	30–60
Minute ventilation (ml/kg/min)	170–350	200–350	NA	NA	100–130	300–400	190–240
Blood volume (ml/kg)	75–90	45–65	70–100	57–60	60–70	50–70	55–65

Notes: The following values are common to all species:

ET CO_2 (mmHg)	30–40	PaO_2 (mmHg)	80–100 (room air: F_IO_2 = .21)
SpO_2 (%)	>95%		>300 (100% oxygen: F_IO_2 = 1.0)
Arterial pH	7.35–7.45	Bicarbonate (mEq/L)	17–25 (small animals)
			25–31 (large animals)
$PaCO_2$ (mmHg)	35–45	Base excess (mEq/L)	−4–+4

* Rates tend to be higher in neonates.

Table 6–4 Troubleshooting Identified Problems During Anesthetic Monitoring

Complication	Potential Causes	Management
Tachypnea	Too light or too deeply anesthetized	Assess anesthetic depth
	Hypoxemia, hypercarbia, acidosis	Assess arterial pH and blood gas
	Hyperthermia	Assess temperature
	Drug induced (opioids, halothane)	Assess compliance, depth
	Atelectasis, pneumothorax, pleural effusion	Aspirate pleural space if indicated
Decreased respiratory rate, apnea, change in character	Too deeply anesthetized	Assess anesthetic depth
	Pressurization in breathing circuit	Check anesthesia machine
	Tube occlusion	Assure patent ET tube
	Effect of injected anesthetic agents	Provide ventilatory support until spontaneous breathing resumes

	Hypothermia	Assess temperature, decrease depth, provide heat
	Iatrogenic hyperventilation	Allow CO_2 to increase to trigger spontaneous ventilation
Sinus bradycardia: * Dogs: <60–70/min Cats: <90–100/min Horses: <20–25/min Cattle: <40–50/min	Drug-induced (alpha$_2$ agonists, opioids)	Administer anticholinergic agent (Appendix 1)
	Excessive anesthetic depth, hypothermia**	Assess temperature, provide heat, decrease anesthetic depth, administer anticholinergic agent
Sm. Ruminants: <50/min	Hypertension, increased ICP Surgically induced vagal stimulation	Ocular and visceral manipulation: stop manipulation
	Hypotension, myocardial ischemia	Assess ABP, oxygenation status
	Hyperkalemia	Review history; assess serum [K+]

(continues)

Table 6–4 *(Continued)*

Complication	Potential Causes	Management
Sinus tachycardia	Too lightly anesthetized (pain)	Assess anesthetic depth
	Hypotension	Assess pulse quality/ABP
		Provide inotropic support
		Assess arterial blood gases
	Hypercapnia, hypoxemia	
	Drug induced (anticholinergic, dissociative agents; thiobarbiturates, catecholamines)	
Hypotension	Too deeply anesthetized	Assess/reduce anesthesia depth†
	Blood or fluid loss	Increase fluid administration rate
		Provide blood/colloid support
	Endotoxemia, sepsis	Review history, provide inotropic support: dobutamine (2–10 mcg or µg/kg/min); dopamine (5–10 mcg or µg/kg/min); ephedrine (0.03–0.1 mg/kg IV bolus, lower dose range for large animals)

Ventricular arrhythmias (PVCs)	Primary myocardial disease/ trauma	Review history; treat when PVCs meet listed criteria
	Hypovolemia, hypotension Hypercapnia, hypoxemia	Assess fluid requirements; ABP Assess arterial blood gas, provide ventilation as indicated
	Inadequate anesthetic depth (pain) Electrolyte imbalances	Assess depth; supplement anesthesia as needed Review history; assess serum electrolyte concentrations
	Criteria for PVC treatment: >15–20/min, multifocal, occurrence in runs, accompanied by poor pulse quality	Lidocaine therapy: 1–2 mg/kg (0.2–0.5 mg/kg for cats, horses): bolus IV 2–4 times over 20 min. For repeated return of PVCs: Start infusion at 50–100 mcg or μg/kg/min (add 1 mg/ml to crystalloid fluid; give at 0.05–0.1 ml/kg/min)

(continues)

ICP = intracranial pressure
ABP = arterial blood pressure

Table 6–4 *(Continued)*

*Guidelines for heart rate are for adults. A higher value should be considered as "minimum" heart rate in neonates. Neonates are more dependent on heart rate for adequate cardiac output, and in general, bradycardia should be treated more aggressively with anticholinergic agent support.

**Animals with profound hypothermia may not respond effectively to anticholinergic agents. Decreasing anesthesia depth and attempts to rewarm are important aspects of management.

†Administration of intraoperative opioids may help to spare general anesthetic requirements with minimal effect on myocardial contractility.

7

Supportive Care During Anesthesia

Supportive care during general anesthesia contributes significantly to a successful outcome. Many factors, such as increased patient risk and prolonged, complex, and invasive procedures, increase the critical need for supportive measures that will assure patient homeostasis during the anesthetic period. Supportive care begins preoperatively with a thorough patient evaluation, including physical examination and appropriate diagnostic evaluation and correction of any abnormalities identified, especially fluid and electrolyte deficits and pH abnormalities. Intraoperative support includes appropriate fluid administration, assurance of acid-base balance, ventilatory support (Chapter 5), administration of adjunct drugs as indicated, provision of external heat, and positioning considerations. The most critical factor guiding supportive care during the anesthetic period is adequate monitoring (Chapter 6). Monitoring is the link between recognition of developing problems and rapid correction before the problem becomes life threatening.

Fluid Therapy

Fluid therapy usually is unnecessary for short procedures in healthy patients, although it is always advisable to have intravenous access established for any anesthetized patient, in case of unexpected blood loss, the need for cardiorespiratory supportive drugs, or additional injectable anesthetic agents. For high-risk patients undergoing invasive, prolonged procedures, fluid administration provides replacement for intraoperative evaporative losses and third space losses associated with surgical trauma or the existing primary disease process, and it helps maintain cardiovascular stability and organ perfusion, which are altered by anesthetic agents.

Most commonly and for most species, a balanced crystalloid fluid similar in composition to extracellular fluid (e.g., LRS or Normosol-R) is administered at a rate of *10 ml/kg/hr.* After the initial two hours of anesthesia, if blood loss is minimal and arterial pressure stable, decreasing the fluid rate to 4–8 ml/kg/hr is recommended to avoid excessive dilution of packed cell volume (PCV) and total protein, especially during prolonged procedures. These fluid rate guidelines must be adjusted, based on the individual patient, blood or other body fluid loss (e.g., third space loss), and blood pressure monitoring, to assure adequate tissue perfusion. Normal body water percentage and distribution and electrolyte composition of body water and several commercially available fluids are listed in Table 7–1.

The following guidelines are for fluid therapy in the perioperative period:

1. Abnormalities identified on preoperative evaluation, including dehydration and acid-base and electrolyte imbalances, should be corrected prior to induction of anesthesia, whenever possible. Table 7–2 provides a general guide for clinical and laboratory assessment of dehydration.

2. Fluids that do not contain an alkalinizing agent (i.e., 0.9% saline, 5% dextrose, Ringer's) tend to promote metabolic acidosis (by dilution) if used for prolonged periods.

3. Blood loss may be replaced with crystalloid fluids at three times the estimated blood volume as long as PCV remains above 20%. This guideline is based on the fact that crystalloid fluids distribute to the entire extracellular fluid volume (ECF), which is approximately three times the blood volume.

4. Fluids to which glucose has been added (for 2.5%, add 25 mg/ml; for 5%, add 50 mg/ml) should be administered to neonates, small patients (<2 kg),

Table 7-1 Body Water Compartment Percentages, the Electrolyte Composition of Body Water, and Commonly Used Parenteral Fluids

	Percentage (% × BW in kg yields L)	Electrolyte Composition (mEq/L)						
		Na	Cl	K	HCO$_3$*	Ca^{+2}	MG^{+2}	Osm**
Body water space								
Total body water	60% (60–75%: higher in neonates; lower with obesity)							
ECF (extracellular fluid)	20–30%							
Plasma volume	5%	142	106	5	24	5	2	282
Blood volume	8–10% (depends on hematocrit)							
Interstitial fluid	15–25% (ECF–plasma volume)	145	115	4	30	3	2	
ICF (intracellular fluid)	30–40%	13	2	155	10	2	2	35

Commercial fluids

LRS	130	109	4	28	3	0	272
Ringer's	147	156	4	0	5	0	312
Normosol-R	148	98	5	27(a) 23(g)	5	0	296
Multisol-R	140	98	5	27(a) 23(g)	3	3	294
5% dextrose (5 gm /dl glucose)	0	0	0	0	0	0	252
0.9% saline	154	154	0	0	0	0	308
Hypertonic saline (7%)	1200	1200	0	0	0	0	2400
1.3% $NaHCO_3$	156	0	0	156	0	0	312
5% $NaHCO_3$	600	0	0	600	0	0	1200
8.4% $NaHCO_3$ (1 mEq/L)	1000	0	0	1000	0	0	2000

*Or bicarbonate-like precursor: LRS (lactate); Normosol-R, or Multisol-R (acetate [a] or gluconate [gl]).

**mOsmol/L.

Table 7–2 Clinical and Laboratory Assessment of Dehydration

% Dehydration*	Skin Tent	MM Moisture	Eye	CRT	PCV**(%)	TP** (gm/dl)
5–6%	2–3 sec	Moist but sticky	Bright, slightly sunken	<3 sec	40–60	7.0–8.0
7–9%	3–5 sec	Sticky to dry	Dull, sunken	3–4 sec	60–65	8.0–9.0
>9%	>5 sec	Dry, cyanotic	Cornea dry	>4 sec	>65%	>9.0

Note: Fluid requirements for dehydration are calculated by the equation

Fluid to administer (L) = % dehydration × body weight (kg)

When time permits, it is best to replace fluid deficit slowly, over 12–24 hr to allow whole body redistribution.

MM = mucous membrane

CRT = capillary refill time

PCV = packed cell volume

TP = total protein

*≤5% dehydration is not clinically detectable.

**Normal PCV and TP values vary among species (Table 1–3) and will be affected by underlying conditions that affect normal values, such as anemia and hypoproteinemia.

avian patients, and animals at risk for hypoglycemia (e.g., those with insulinoma, diabetes mellitus, portal caval shunt) to avoid a hypoglycemic crisis. It is advisable to monitor blood glucose levels during prolonged anesthetic periods.

5. Administration of large quantities of fluids at room temperature can contribute significantly to hypothermia. Efforts should be taken to warm fluids (cocooning the administration line in hot water bottles, warming the fluids, using commercially available infusion warmers during prolonged administration; Figure 7–1), especially in small patients.

6. Administration of large quantities of fluids can contribute to the development of cerebral and pulmonary edema (this depends on many factors, including fluid administration rate, patient's serum protein concentration, and cardiac function). In at-risk patients, consider administration of a colloid, if necessary, to maintain adequate circulating volume and blood pressure.

7. Animals that may not handle volume overload (e.g., those with mitral insufficiency) should receive fluids at 50% or less the standard rate.

8. Maximum rate of fluid administration is 90 ml/kg/hr for most domestic species; cats should not receive greater than 50 ml/kg/hr. Higher rates (up to 360 ml/kg/hr) probably will be tolerated in relatively healthy patients; administer fluids as rap-

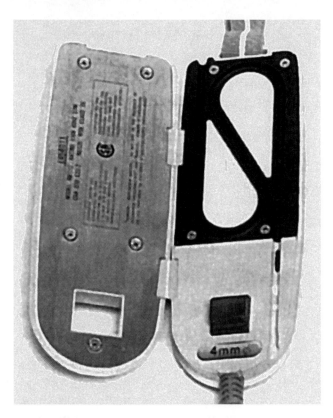

Figure 7–1 Infusion warmers are available in two sizes to accommodate fluid and blood administration sets. These devices are especially useful for administering blood products or large volumes of fluid during prolonged procedures to help minimize hypothermia. (Reprinted with permission from Thurmon et al., eds., *Lumb and Jones' Veterinary Anesthesia*, 3rd ed., Baltimore: Williams & Wilkins, 1996, page 579.)

idly as necessary to achieve hemodynamic stability and decrease the rate as soon as this occurs.

9. For hypokalemic animals, it is best to correct the deficit prior to anesthesia; K^+-supplemented fluids administered during anesthesia could result in cardiac conduction disturbances, if fluid administration were suddenly increased. Potassium supplementation is common (adding 10–30 mEq/L) during supportive care of patients with a variety of abnormalities, such as anorexia, diarrhea, or vomiting. Intravenous potassium administration must not exceed 0.5 mEq/kg/hr.

10. Intraoperative serial assessment of packed cell volume and total protein is advisable in prolonged procedures and necessary when significant blood loss occurs. While numbers vary in the literature, blood loss greater than 20% of total blood volume (i.e., 8–10% of body weight; Table 6–3) in healthy patients and greater than 10% loss in critical patients should be replaced with whole blood, packed red cells, or an artificial blood solution, depending on availability. Colloids should be administered when hypoproteinemia is present or when crystalloid fluids fail to maintain adequate blood pressure (i.e., minimum of 60 mmHg, mean arterial pressure). Table 7–3 lists some available blood and colloid products and basic indications and guidelines for use.

Table 7-3 Adjuncts to Fluid Therapy During Anesthesia: Indications, Side Effects, and General Guidelines for Use

Product	Indications	Side Effects	Dosage/Comments
Blood replacements			
Whole blood*	Anemia, hemorrhage	Immune reaction cross-match is recommended especially with repeat transfusions	1. Based on estimated loss 2. Based on equation: $$\text{Amount} = \frac{\text{desired PCV} - \text{actual PCV}}{\text{donor PCV}} \times \text{recipient blood volume}$$ 3. Empirical: 10–40 ml/kg (dog) and 5–20 ml/kg (cats), frequent reassessment
Packed red cells**	Anemia, hemorrhage	Same as previous	Same as previous. Dilute with saline to administer.
Blood substitute†	Anemia, hemorrhage	Urine/tissue discoloration, volume overload, arrythmias, *renal toxicity*	15–30 ml/kg: *rate <10 ml/ kg/hr*

Colloids		
Plasma*	Hypoproteinemia, Allergic reaction, volume overload	10–20 ml/kg, initial empirical dose. Calculation may be based on the equation: $$\text{Amount} = \frac{\text{desired TP} - \text{actual TP}}{\text{donor plasma TP}}$$ $$\times \text{ recipient plasma volume}$$ End point directed by serial TP assessment. Intravascular life-span: 4–15 days
Dextran (40 and 70)	Same as for plasma	5–20 ml/kg over 24 hr (more rapid for shock) End point is directed by stabilization of ABP. Intravascular life-span: 2–24 hr
Hetastarch	Same as for plasma, coagulopathy	5–20 ml/kg over 24 hr (more rapid for shock) End point is directed by stabilization of ABP.

(continues)

Table 7-3 *(Continued)*

Product	Indications	Side Effects	Dosage/Comments
			Intravascular life-span: 6 hr (longer for Pentastarch)
Alkalinizing agents			
Bicarbonate	Metabolic acidosis	Intracellular acidosis	1. Administer if pH <7.2 or base deficit is >−10 mEq/L. Avoid in the presence of hypoventilation because hypercapnia is exacerbated and pH further decreased by increased formation of CO_2 when HCO_3 combines with H^+ ions. Do not coadminister with Ca^{++} or blood products. 2. Quantity to administer is based on base deficit. Quantity (mEq/L) = Base deficit × 0.3 × body

Tromethamine organic amine buffer (0.3 M)	Metabolic acidosis	weight (kg). Give 1/4–1/2 of calculated deficit over 30 min and reassess.
		1. Dosage (ml) = base deficit × 1.1 × body weight (kg)
		2. Administer slowly; rapid infusion can cause ECG changes similar to hyperkalemia.
		3. Administration is contraindicated with uremia and anuria.
Cardiovascular drugs		
Lidocaine	Osmotic diuresis, hypoglycemia increases coagulation times	
	Ventricular arrhythmias, ventricular tachycardia	See criteria in text Dosages listed in Table 6–4. Avoid when heart rate is low (<120–140/min for dogs); it may induce profound bradycardia and have significant negative effect on cardiac output.

(continues)

Table 7-3 *(Continued)*

Product	Indications	Side Effects	Dosage/Comments
Dobutamine	Hypotension	Sinus tachycardia, arrhythmias	2–10 µg/kg/minute
Dopamine	Hypotension, decreased urine production	Sinus tachycardia, arrhythmias	5–10 µg/kg/min: low dose (2–5 µg/kg/min) is recommended for increasing renal perfusion to improve urine formation.
Ephedrine	Hypotension	Sinus tachycardia	0.03–0.1 mg/kg IV bolus: lower dose range for large animals. Reported to spare uterine blood flow, which may be particularly beneficial for pregnant patients.
Epinephrine	Refractory hypotension	*Arrhythmias* Sinus tachycardia	0.01–0.03 µg/kg/min Contraindicated during halothane anesthesia

| Isoproterenol | Bradycardia | Arrhythmias, hypotension (B_2 effect) | 0.01–0.1 µg/kg/min |

Note: Blood and plasma must be administered through in-line filter to remove clots and cellular debris. Blood should not be mixed with calcium- or bicarbonate-containing fluids.

Fresh whole blood and *fresh frozen* plasma also are effective in treating coagulopathy, including von Willebrand's disease. The former also is effective in treatment of thrombocytopenia. The latter also is effective in treating platelet dysfunction and specific clotting factor deficits.

**Packed cells are better for anemia *not* accompanied by hypovolemia, while whole blood or packed cells plus colloid are better for acute (significant) hemorrhage.

†Several products exist, including free-hemoglobin-based, liposome-encapsulated hemoglobin and perflurorocarbons; and one product, Oxyglobin™ (free-hemoglobin based), currently is approved for use in veterinary medicine.

11. Metabolic acidosis may be preexisting or develop during anesthesia due to poor perfusion or hypothermia and may require treatment in some cases. Alkalinizing agents should be considered if the pH is <7.2 and the acidosis is due to the metabolic component (i.e., PCO_2 is within normal limits; see the acid-base section later).

Routes of Administration

While subcutaneous fluid replacement with isotonic fluid (preferably without dextrose or at concentrations ≤2.5%) is acceptable for mild dehydration, moderate to severe dehydration requiring relatively rapid correction should be treated with intravenous fluids. While venous access usually is no problem in most species under relatively normal conditions, neonates and severely volume-depleted animals can present a challenge. For very small and very hypotensive patients or patients with thrombosed peripheral vasculature, the intraosseous route of fluid administration may provide the necessary access to reestablish fluid balance prior to and during anesthesia. This route also is effective for infusion of a variety of anesthetic agents and cardiosupportive drugs. The most common access sites in small animals include the medial surface of the proximal tibia 1–2 cm distal to the tibial tuberosity, the tibial tuberosity, the trocanteric fossa of the femur, the wing of the ilium, the ischium, and the greater tubercle of the humerus. In birds, access sites include the distal ulna and the proximal tibiotarsus (see Figure 11–2). A spinal needle (20–22 ga) is preferred if patient size will accommodate placement. Hypodermic needles (22–25 ga) are more appropriate for very small patients, but these have a tendency to become blocked with a bone piece during entry through the cortex. The needles are placed aseptically, capped, and utilized like IV catheters; they usually are sewn or taped to the skin using a tape butterfly and protected with a bulky wrap to prevent bending or breaking. Fluid rate is limited to 11 ml/min and can be doubled using pressurization (300 mmHg). Contraindications for intraosseous cannulation include recent fractures, pneumatic bones, infection over the access site, and sepsis.

Acid-Base Balance

Normal blood pH (7.35–7.45) is maintained through three general mechanisms: *buffer systems* (bicarbonate is the major extracellular buffer, where pH = 6.1 + log $HCO_3^-/H_2CO_3^-$; hemoglobin, plasma protein, and phosphate play a lesser role) cushion insults that alter the pH; the *lungs* (respiratory mechanism) alter the pH through changes in PCO_2 (normal $PaCO_2$ = 35–45 mmHg; hypoventilation will increase $PaCO_2$, and hyperventilation will decrease $PaCO_2$); and the *kidney* (metabolic mechanism) affects the pH through excretion of H^+ and generation and resorption of HCO_3^- (normal: HCO_3^- = 17–31 mEq/L).

The acid-base status should be assessed prior to anesthetic induction in high-risk patients. If preexisting metabolic disorders are identified, anesthesia should be postponed until the disorders are corrected, as general anesthesia can exacerbate an acid-base imbalance. Disorders of the pH can affect electrolyte concentrations (the pH affects potassium concentration inversely: decreased pH $\Rightarrow$ increased K^+ and vice versa; pH affects ionized calcium inversely: decreased pH $\Rightarrow$ increased ionized Ca^{++} and vice versa), cardiac contractility, vascular responsiveness, and normal cellular function.

Four primary disturbances in pH balance can occur (Table 7–4), and the complexity of interpretation is increased by compensatory responses (the opposing system responds to turn pH back toward the normal range) and the potential for a mixed disorder in some patients.

Oxygenation

Arterial oxygen tension (PaO_2), included in routine arterial blood gas analysis, provides accurate assessment of the patient's ability to oxygenate the blood and provide adequate tissue oxygenation during anesthesia. Tissue oxygenation is determined by hemoglobin concentration, hemoglobin saturation (SpO_2, which is determined by PaO_2; Figure 6–2A), and blood delivery (cardiac output as reflected by arterial blood pressure). *Five factors contribute to decreased arterial oxygen tension (PaO_2):*

Table 7–4 Alterations in, Causes of, and Compensatory Mechanisms Involved in Acid-Base Balance

Primary Disorder/ Compensatory Response	Noncompensated			Compensated**			Causes
	pH	PCO$_2$	HCO$_3$*	pH	PCO$_2$	HCO$_3$	
Respiratory acidosis/ metabolic alkalosis	↓↓	↑	↑	↓	↑	↑↑	Anesthesia, obesity, thoracic or brain disease
Respiratory alkalosis/ metabolic acidosis	↑↑	↓	↓	↑	↓	↓↓	Iatrogenic, excessive IPPV, fever, hypoxemia, anxiety
Metabolic acidosis/ respiratory alkalosis	↓↓	N	↓	↓	↓	↓	Poor perfusion, shock, renal disease, ketoacidosis, diarrhea
Metabolic alkalosis/ respiratory acidosis	↑↑	N	↑	↑	↑	↑	Acute vomiting, upper GI obstruction (ruminants), hypokalemia

(continues)

Table 7-4 (Continued)

Note: Two acid-base disturbances can occur independently (e.g. trauma resulting in shock and severe pulmonary hemorrhage resulting in metabolic and respiratory acidosis) with increased severity in the pH changes, or, in the case of two opposing independent disorders (metabolic alkalosis associated with upper GI obstruction with anesthetic-induced respiratory depression), can exist with a near normal pH. Knowledge of the case history and laboratory findings will help to discern compensatory response versus two primary disorders.

During anesthesia, correction of respiratory-induced pH changes involves an appropriate change in ventilatory support. Metabolic acidosis is best corrected prior to anesthesia. Treatment with bicarbonate should be considered if the base excess value (normal values are listed in Table 6–3) is greater than −10 mEq/L and only if normal $PaCO_2$ values are established. Bicarbonate dosage in mEq/L = Base excess value × BW (kg) × 0.3.

Give approximately one fourth the dose and reassess blood gas analysis. Repeat until pH and base excess return to normal limits. Metabolic alkalosis is treated by administration of bicarbonate-free fluids (e.g., 0.9% saline).

*HCO_3 increases with respiratory acidosis and decreases with respiratory alkalosis by approximately 1–2 mEq/L for each 10 mmHg change in PCO_2, according to the equation:

$$CO_2 + H_2O \rightleftarrows H_2CO_3 \rightleftarrows HCO_3^- + H^+$$

**As a general rule, the compensatory response occurs when the primary disturbance becomes chronic and acts to bring the blood pH back *toward* (but usually not completely into) the normal range, which helps differentiate primary from compensatory changes. Compensatory respiratory mechanisms are maximal within 8–12 hr. Compensatory metabolic mechanisms are maximal within 3–5 days and more effective (than respiratory) in returning the pH to normal.

decreased inspired concentration (F_IO_2), hypoventilation, diffusion abnormality, ventilation-perfusion (VQ) mismatch, and right-to-left shunt. All but the last benefit from enriched oxygen delivery (F_IO_2 = 1.0 or 100% versus room air; F_IO_2 = 0.21 or 21%). Anesthetized patients are susceptible to hypoventilation and VQ mismatch, especially horses, and supplemental oxygen is recommended in all patients, especially those at increased risk for development of hypoxemia (e.g., those with respiratory abnormalities). Hypoxemia is defined as PaO_2 <60 mmHg (which corresponds approximately to SpO_2 = 90%). The PaO_2 value should be maintained *at least* above 60 mmHg and preferably above 100 mmHg throughout the perianesthetic period.

Intraoperative Adjunct Drugs

The use of various agents to support cardiac performance during general anesthesia is guided by the monitoring devices applied during the anesthetic period. Continuous electrocardiography detects rhythm disturbances that might benefit from therapeutic intervention, and quantitative blood pressure monitoring (either invasive or noninvasive) guides the need for inotropic support. *Ventricular premature complexes* should be treated *if* they are multiform, appear to be superimposed on the previous T wave, occur in runs, are >15–20/min in frequency, or have a significant detrimental effect on arterial blood pressure. Lidocaine dosages are listed in

Table 6–4. Ventricular tachycardia may respond to lidocaine *if* a pulse is present and the rate is ≥150/minute.

Hypotension not responsive to fluid bolus and decreasing the depth of anesthesia may benefit from inotropic agent administration. Dobutamine and dopamine must be administered as an infusion due to their short duration of effect. Ephedrine, as an IV bolus, will provide blood pressure support by both direct and indirect effects at both alpha and beta receptors; the effects may persist for 10–30 min. Dosages are listed in Table 6–4. An ECG should be monitored during administration, as these agents can promote arrhythmias. Infusion of epinephrine has been suggested for hypotension that fails to respond to the more commonly used inotropes. Due to its inherent arrhythmogenicity, epinephrine should be reserved for refractory cases and avoided during halothane anesthesia.

Prevention of Hypothermia

Hypothermia occurs commonly during general anesthesia, especially in small and neonatal patients, due to the relatively large body surface to mass ratio and contributing factors including inhalation of dry, cold anesthetic gases; contact with cold surfaces; wet skin from surgical site preparation; exposure of body cavities during the procedure; anesthetic-induced vasodilation; and thermoregulatory depression. Severe hypothermia can cause brain damage, ventilatory depression, life-threatening cardiac arrhythmias and conduction disturbances, and acid-base and electrolyte derangements, which contribute significantly to delayed recoveries. Several methods are available to limit heat loss during anesthesia, including maintaining the ambient temperature between 21 and 25°C, keeping the patient on a circulating water blanket, applying "space" wraps or forced air blanket heaters when possible, and using warmed intravenous crystalloid fluids when relatively large quantities are administered. Minimizing anesthesia time is one of the most critical factors in the prevention of severe hypothermia. Monitoring the patient's temperature with an esophageal probe to assess the core temperature is the most accurate representation of the patient's heat balance. Small patients benefit from recovery in incubators, if available. Measures to facilitate return to normothermia during recovery include providing a warm ambient temperature, using water-circulating blankets to "cocoon" the patient, using heat lamps, and administering warm IV fluids, if therapy is continued into the postoperative period. As patients recover, shivering invariably occurs as part of the warming process and can increase oxygen consumption fivefold, often at a time when respiration still is depressed. Providing supplemental oxygen until the body temperature has returned to near normal helps prevent development of hypoxemia and is especially important in high-risk patients, such as those with underlying respiratory or cardiac abnormalities. Temperature monitoring should be continued until the temperature returns to normal. To avoid hyperthermia, it is advisable to remove heating devices once the body temperature reaches 98–99°F and the patient is awake and showing spontaneous movement.

Positioning Considerations

Padding and positioning are of greater concern in large animal patients, but some considerations for positioning small animal patients deserve mention. Considerations for both large and small patients assume even greater importance during prolonged procedures. Tilting patients to a "head-down" position, as for ovariohysterectomy, has minimal adverse effects in the short term and in healthy patients but should be avoided for prolonged periods and in high-risk patients due to respiratory compromise. Positioning the forelimbs forward is common and not detrimental if done loosely. However, extreme extension of the forelimbs can interfere with respiratory movement and cause brachial neuropathy if applied for long periods of time. The dependent lung (lateral recumbency) becomes atelectic over time, and this effect is exacerbated with duration of anesthesia. In patients with unilateral lung disease, it is beneficial to place the more "normal" lung up, when possible. Assure that the airway stays patent by keeping the neck and head slightly extended and assure unrestricted respiratory movement (equipment and elbows should not be placed on the thoracic area).

Large animal patients should be placed on a padded surface to minimize the risk of postanesthetic myopathy—this is *essential* for equine patients during gas anesthesia. Available padding includes bags that can be filled with air once the animal is positioned (dunnage bags) and thick (4 in. minimum) foam- or water-filled pads. Laterally recumbent animals should have the lower forelimb extended forward to minimize the risk of entrapping the brachial plexus with resultant neuropathy. The upper limbs should be supported to maintain them parallel to the table surface (see additional species-specific recommendations in species chapters). These considerations are of lesser importance in small ruminants and camelids, but padding (2 in. minimum) should be provided for these patients.

8

Pain Management

The definition, recognition, and management of pain has become a central issue in veterinary practice due to increased awareness and knowledge by veterinarians and pet owners. Pain is an unpleasant sensory or emotional experience associated with actual or potential tissue damage and has been described as "an experience for which there is no direct measure." Pain causes distress and suffering, which contributes greatly to the stress associated with hospitalization and anesthesia. A series of behavioral, physiologic, endocrine, metabolic, and cellular responses accompany pain, which maintain and amplify the pain response. Except to warn that something is wrong, pain rarely, if ever, has beneficial effects, and unmanaged pain interferes with normal behavior patterns. Activation of the sympathetic nervous system secondary to pain may result in protein catabolism, abnormal renal function, electrolyte disturbances, immune suppression, and delayed healing.

Pain is difficult to quantitate because many animals are stoic; and signs of pain vary greatly with species, breed, age, health status, behavioral patterns, and pain intensity. Table 8–1 lists physiologic and behavioral signs that may be (but are not exclusively) associated with pain as well as some specific painful insults and the expected degree of associated pain. Because signs of pain are often nonspecific and sometimes discrete, management of pain in veterinary patients often is inadequate. It is important to maintain a liberal attitude regarding analgesic therapy. While overtreatment may occur, the consequences of unnecessary analgesia and side effects must be weighed against the detrimental effects of unrelieved pain. In general, any procedure known to be painful in humans should be assumed to be painful in animals and treated appropriately.

Physiology of Pain

Nociceptive signals are transmitted to the spinal cord by fine myelinated A-delta fibers and unmyelinated C fibers, with their cell bodies contained in the dorsal root ganglia. Two neuron types have been identified: nociceptive specific neurons (which respond to input from discrete

Table 8–1 Physiologic and Behavioral Signs That May Be Associated with Pain and Some Examples of Painful Insults and the Expected Degree of Associated Pain

Physiologic Signs*	Behavioral Signs	Painful Insult/Degree of Pain**
Tachypnea	Vocalization	Surgery†: mild, moderate, severe
Tachycardia	Restlessness	*Mild to moderate surgical pain:*
Hypertension	Agitation	Castration, ovariohysterectomy, exploratory
Dilated pupils	Abnormal posturing	Laparotomy, onychectomy
Salivation	Personality change	*Severe to distressing surgical pain:*
Pale mucous membranes	Anorexia	Amputations, orthopedic procedures, thoracotomies,
Cardiac arrhythmias	Decreased grooming	Spinal surgery, auricular surgery, perianal surgery
Hyperglycemia	Excessive licking or chewing	Trauma—mild to distressing
	Oblivious to surroundings	Pancreatitis—distressing
		Peritonitis—distressing

*Many signs may be difficult to differentiate from effects of anesthetic emergence and drugs administered during the anesthetic period especially in the immediate postoperative period.

**Degree of pain associated with a specific insult varies greatly with individual animal and surgical technique.

†Surgical pain is divided into the three categories, with more invasive procedures and more extensive tissue trauma causing greater pain.

topographical areas) and wide dynamic range neurons (which respond to a wide range of stimuli). It is believed that the latter type is more important in nociception and responsible for central sensitization of receptive fields with long-term activation of afferent pathways, which has been referred to as *wind up*. This mechanism is believed to be due to repeated C-fiber stimulation, which leads to continued release of neurotransmitters that facilitate nociception (e.g., substance P, glutamic acid, N-methyl-D-aspartate [NMDA], neurotensin, cholecystokinin). Once activated, transmission of afferent signals to higher brain centers, including the thalamic, medullary, pontine, and cortical regions, occurs via the spinothalamic, spinocervical, spinomesencephalic, and spinoreticular tracts.

Pain perception is a complex process that may be modified clinically at several sites, including reduction of afferent input (local techniques), signal integration and transmission (regional techniques), or integration and recognition at higher centers (parenterally administered agents). Analgesic administration *before* the onset of pain (preemptive analgesia) provides better control of pain in the postoperative period. Combining agents that act at different sites (multimodal therapy) may provide superior pain management for both acute and refractory pain with fewer side effects. With these considerations in mind, the following agents and techniques provide several options for pain management.

Therapeutic Options

Agents for pain management may be administered on a scheduled basis or dictated by dynamic patient assessment. Available drugs for analgesia include the opioids and alpha$_2$ agonists, applied epidurally or parenterally; local anesthetic agents; ketamine; and nonsteroidal anti-inflammatory agents (NSAIDs).

Opioids

Opioid agonists and agonist-antagonists are effective in the management of acute moderate to severe pain and also provide variable degrees of sedation. Opioids are classified according to the specific opioid receptor that they modulate, vary in their analgesic and sedative properties, and are scheduled according to their potential for addiction (Appendix 2). Pure agonists, including morphine, oxymorphone, hydromorphone, meperidine, and fentanyl, provide analgesia with variable durations of action (Table 8–2). Side effects include dose-dependent respiratory depression and a vagomimetic effect, which promotes bradycardia. Myocardial contractility is well-maintained with opioids.

Morphine and meperidine may cause histamine release, resulting in hypotension, when administered intravenously (IV); therefore, the subcutaneous or intramuscular routes are preferred. The short duration of action and low potency of meperidine makes it less

Table 8-2 Dosages of Analgesic Agents in Dogs and Cats

	Dose (mg/kg)		Route	Duration (hr)	Comments
	Dog	Cat			
Systemic opioids					
Morphine	0.05–0.6	0.05–0.2	IM, SC	2–6	Use with tranquilizer (cats)
SR (sustained-release)	1.0–3.0	—	PO	12	
Oxymorphone	0.05–0.2	0.05–0.1	IM, SC, IV	2–6	Use with tranquilizer (cats), 4 mg max dose
Hydromorphone	0.1–0.2	0.05–0.1	IM, SC	2–4	Use with tranquilizer (cats)
Meperidine	1.0–4.0	1.0–3.0	IM, SC	0.51	
Fentanyl	25 μg (<10 kg) 50 μg (10–20 kg) 75 μg (20–30 kg)		Trans-dermal	Up to 72	12–24 hr onset of effect (anecdotal reports of dysphoria in both species)

	100 µg (>30 kg) 2–6 µg/kg bolus	2–6 µg/kg/min (same) 2–6 µg/kg/hr	IV IV	<1 (prior to CRI) CRI	
Butorphanol	0.1–0.4	0.1–0.4	IM, SC, IV	1–3	
Buprenorphine	0.005–0.02	0.005–0.01	IM, SC, IV	4–8	
Epidural opioids					
Morphine	0.1	0.1		10–20	Dilute with saline (1 ml/5 kg) *Or use* Bupivacaine (1 ml/5 kg) (6 ml max. volume has been recommended)
Oxymorphone	0.1	0.1		10	

(continues)

Table 8–2 *(Continued)*

	Dose (mg/kg)				
	Dog	**Cat**	**Route**	**Duration (hr)**	**Comments**
Fentanyl	0.004	0.004		<1	
Butorphanol	0.25	0.25		2–4	
Buprenorphine	0.003–0.005	0.003–0.005		12–18	
Intra-articular opioids					
Morphine	0.1 mg/kg in 0.5 ml/kg bupivacaine	–		12–24	
*Systemic alpha$_2$ agonists**					
Xylazine	0.01–0.2	0.01–0.2	IM, SC, IV	1–3	
Medetomidine	0.002–0.01	0.002–0.01	IM, SC, IV	1–4	

Epidural alpha$_2$ agonists					
Xylazine	0.2	0.2		1–3	
Medetomidine	0.01	0.01		4	
Ketamine (with diazepam, equal volume)	0.25	0.25	IV	1–2	
	0.2	0.2	IV		
Infusion					
Loading dose	0.25–0.5 mg/kg	Same	IV	—	
Intraoperative	10 µg/kg/min	Same	IV	—	
Recovery	2 µg/kg/min	Same	IV	≤ 24 hr	Requires continuous observation
Nonsteroidal anti-inflammatory drugs					
Carprofen**	2.0–4.0	2.0	PO	24	One dose only (cats)
	2.0–4.0	2.0	IV, SC	24	One dose only (both)
Etodolac	10–15	—	PO	24	
Ketoprofen	0.5–1.0	0.5–1.0	PO	24	One dose only (both)

(continues)

Table 8-2 *(Continued)*

	Dose (mg/kg)				
	Dog	Cat	Route	Duration (hr)	Comments
Aspirin	10–25	10–15	PO	8–12 (dog) 24 (cat)	
Phenylbutazone	10–25	10–15	PO	8–12	Limited use (both)
Meloxicam**	0.1–0.2 PO and SC	0.1–0.3 PO only	PO	24	0.2 SC (or 0.3 PO) for first dose, then 0.1 PO; 4 days max (cats)
Naproxen	1.0–2.0	–	PO	24	
Piroxicam	0.2–0.4	–	PO	48	
Flunixin meglumine	0.5–1.0	–	IM, IV		One dose only
Acetaminophen	10–15	–	PO	12	

Note: See species-specific chapters for recommendations for horses, ruminants, swine, birds, reptiles, and small mammals.

CRI = constant rate infusion

*Do not use alpha$_2$ agonists in high-risk patients.

**Injectable carprofen is not currently available in the United States. Meloxicam is not currently available in the United States.

useful than other opioids. Fentanyl is a potent agonist with a short duration of effect. It is available for transdermal application in four sizes and for IV use as repeated bolus or constant rate infusion (see Table 8–2). The latter use requires constant patient observation but is very effective in acute, severe pain management. Opioid agonists can cause dysphoria in cats, but concurrent use of a tranquilizer (a benzodiazepine or acepromazine) minimizes this side effect; tranquilizers are also beneficial in dogs when pain relief afforded by an opioid results in increased activity or (rarely) dysphoria. The opioid agonist-antagonist butorphanol provides moderate analgesia and minimal sedation in both dogs and cats and rarely causes excitement in cats. Buprenorphine is a partial opioid agonist, useful for dogs and cats, that provides moderate analgesia and has a duration of action of 6–12 hr. An advantage of the opioids is reversibility with opioid antagonists, including naloxone and nalmefene, should an adverse response occur. Butorphanol may be used to reverse excessive respiratory depression induced by an opioid agonist while preserving some analgesia.

Opioids, including morphine, oxymorphone, fentanyl, butorphanol, and buprenorphine, have been used epidurally to provide analgesia of variable duration (see Table 8–2) while minimizing sedation and the adverse effects that may accompany systemic opioid administration. The technique for epidural injection of opioids is identical to that for local anesthetic agents (described in Chapter 3) and the two are often combined for a more profound and prolonged effect. The advantage of epidural opioids over local anesthetic agents is that motor and sympathetic nerve functions are preserved and duration is longer when morphine, buprenorphine, and oxymorphone are used. Normal rear limb activity is maintained and hypotension secondary to vasodilation, seen with local anesthetics, does not occur. An epidural technique is contraindicated in the presence of bleeding abnormalities, sepsis, or infected skin at the site of injection; epidural administration of local anesthetics is contraindicated for hypovolemic patients.

Alpha$_2$ Agonists

Alpha$_2$ agonists, including xylazine, detomidine (horses), and medetomidine, provide good short-term analgesia and sedation. The side effects of alpha$_2$ agonists are listed in Chapter 2, and these effects are exacerbated by concurrently used anesthetic agents. Due to the cardiovascular effects and the relatively short duration of analgesia, use of these agents for analgesia should be reserved for healthy animals recovering from elective procedures or suffering from relatively minor trauma. Concurrent administration with opioids will enhance the analgesic effect and allow for use of minimal effective dosages. Alpha$_2$ agonists are reversible with alpha$_2$ antagonists, including yohimbine, atipamezole, and tolazoline (see Table 8–2). Both xylazine and medetomidine (and detomidine in horses and swine; see Tables 3–4 and 3–5) have been used epidurally. While of lesser concern in horses and swine, the potential for systemic side effects and the relatively short duration of action make them less useful than the opioids in small animals, with one advantage being easy accessibility (not scheduled).

Ketamine

Subanesthetic doses of ketamine have been used in humans for relief of acute and chronic pain. Ketamine provides somatic analgesia in animals and is not recommended as the sole agent for visceral pain management. Undesirable side effects, including dysphoria, seizures, and muscle rigidity, may be minimized by using ketamine in combination with a tranquilizer. Specific contraindications are listed in Chapter 2. Dosages have not been definitively established for pain management in animals, but suggested guidelines are included in Table 8–2.

Nonsteroidal Anti-Inflammatory Agents

NSAIDs are used for the treatment of mild to moderate pain. The side effects are due to inhibition of physiologic (protective) prostaglandins and include gastrointestinal ulceration and renal tubular necrosis. With development of more selective NSAIDs, which are more potent inhibitors of inflammation and less organ toxic, these agents, in combination with an opioid, have been applied for preemptive and perioperative management of acute surgical pain.

Carprofen is a more specific inhibitor of cyclooxygenase-2. It is approved for oral use in dogs in the United States, but cat dosages have been reported (see Table 8–2). While side effects are less likely than from other NSAIDs, gastrointestinal disturbances have been reported and acute hepatopathy has been described.

Etodolac is another specific cyclooxygenase-2 inhibitor with fewer side effects. It is approved for use in dogs in the United States for management of osteoarthritis pain.

Ketoprofen is a relatively new NSAID with potent anti-inflammatory activity but greater potential for side effects than carprofen. It is approved for use in cats and dogs in Europe. Ketoprofen causes gastrointestinal and renal effects at therapeutic doses and should be avoided in high-risk patients and in the preoperative period.

Meloxicam is approved for use in dogs in Europe. It is marketed for treatment of chronic skeletal pain but has been shown to be effective in the management of moderate postoperative pain. Dosages are available for cats; however, data regarding its safety currently are unavailable.

Aspirin is a potent analgesic and anti-inflammatory agent that may be used in both dogs and cats. Gastric ulceration can occur at therapeutic doses with a lesser risk when buffered preparations are used. Dosing frequency is less in the cat due to prolonged plasma elimination.

Use of other NSAIDs, including phenylbutazone, naproxen, piroxicam, and flunixin meglumine, in dogs and cats has been reported and dosages are listed in Table 8–2. *Flunixin* is a potent visceral analgesic that also may modulate the pathophysiologic response to endotoxin. While dosages are available, data supporting the use of these agents are lacking and there is a greater incidence of adverse side effects; therefore, these drugs should not be used unless safer agents are unavailable and the need outweighs the potential for adverse effects.

Acetaminophen is an atypical NSAID with excellent analgesic effects but limited anti-inflammatory activity. Its use in cats is contraindicated due to methemoglobin formation.

Local and Regional Techniques

Application of local anesthetic techniques has been shown to decrease the intensity of postoperative pain. Blocking nociceptive impulse entry into the cord probably prevents development of the sustained hyperexcitable state of the central nervous system largely responsible for sustained postoperative pain. Several local techniques and their applications are described in Chapter 3. Bupivacaine is the local anesthetic of choice for pain management due to duration of effect; suggested dosages for the specific techniques are included in Chapter 3.

Selection of appropriate analgesic drugs and techniques for pain management is influenced by many factors, including the animal's previous behavior pattern; the type, duration, and invasiveness of the procedure or extent and location of the traumatic injury; mental status; and overall patient condition. Like anesthetic management, no one agent or technique is applicable for every situation; however, every case should be assessed and treated according to the preceding considerations.

9

Introduction to Anesthetic Management in Specific Species

Chapters 10–17 provide brief overviews of anesthetic management for a variety of veterinary species, including considerations that might be unique to that particular species, such as restraint, venous access, intubation, positioning, monitoring, and recovery, as well as suggested protocols for premedication, induction, and total parenteral anesthesia. Anesthetic protocols should be formulated to produce the desired result safely, effectively, and economically, based on the patient's temperament, physical status, *a thorough physical examination,* appropriate laboratory and diagnostic tests, and procedure duration and complexity, regardless of species.

A few general statements apply to all species:

1. Endotracheal intubation to preserve and protect a patent airway should be performed for animals undergoing prolonged procedures or for those with unknown fasting status. Intubation is advised, but not essential, in species that do not vomit (horses, rabbits) or present a greater challenge to intubation (rabbits, pigs).

2. The endotracheal tube should be coated lightly with a sterile lubricant prior to insertion to minimize tracheal irritation.

3. Evidence of proper tube placement includes *seeing* the tube pass between the arytenoids (horses and adult cattle are an exception, see Chapters 15 and 16), observing condensation inside the tube with expiration, eliciting a cough when the tube passes into the trachea, and watching the rebreathing bag move with respiration. Air should be placed in the tube cuff only to the point where providing a breath by squeezing the bag (with the relief valve closed) does not result in gases escaping around the tube (smelled or heard). This practice will help to avoid overinflation of the cuff, which can result in damage to the tracheal mucosa. *If* you cannot create an effective seal with cuff inflation or the animal awakens, reassess for proper placement.

4. Eye lubrication should be applied to all anesthetized animals, as general anesthesia obtunds tearing and the ability to blink, so as to maintain a moist cornea.

5. Monitoring may be simple or complex, depending on the length and invasiveness of the procedure. Available techniques (Chapter 6) apply to all veterinary species with some species-specific considerations.

6. As a general rule, anticholinergic agents are not considered a routine part of the preanesthetic protocol in any species but can be used as such in healthy small animals, especially when drugs known to decrease heart rate (e.g., opioids) are part of the protocol. Anticholinergics may precipitate colic in horses, and horses are rarely susceptible to bradycardia during the anesthetic period; therefore, routine perioperative use is contraindicated. Anticholinergic administration will not eliminate ruminant salivation and, in fact, may increase the viscosity of secretions, making them harder to clear; therefore, routine use is not recommended.

10

Anesthetic Management of Dogs

A variety of protocols are available to provide chemical restraint/premedication, induction of anesthesia, and total parenteral anesthesia in dogs (Table 10–1). A neuroleptanalgesic (tranquilizer plus opioid) combination will minimize anxiety and struggling for catheterization, minimize requirements for induction and maintenance agents, and provide preemptive analgesia. Popular and economical combinations are acepromazine with morphine (moderate to severe pain), hydromorphone (moderate to severe pain), or butorphanol (mild to moderate pain).

Diazepam can be substituted for acepromazine when the latter is contraindicated (see Chapter 2). Midazolam provides a convenient (but expensive) alternative

Table 10–1 Recommended Dosages and Protocols for Chemical Restraint, Preanesthetic Protocols, Induction Agents, and Total Parenteral Anesthesia for Dogs

Protocol	Dosages (mg/kg) (IV, IM, SC)*	Comments
Chemical restraint/ premedication		Animals can be aroused during chemical restraint.
Opioid plus**		
Acepromazine or	0.05	Max dose: 2 mg (premed), 4 mg (restraint).
Diazepam or	0.2	Max recommended dose: 10 mg.
Midazolam	0.1–0.2	Max recommended dose: 10 mg.
		Benzodiazepines are preferred for high-risk, neonatal, and geriatric patients.
Morphine	0.4–1.0	Avoid IV route, potential for histamine release.
Oxymorphone	0.1–0.2	
Hydromorphone	0.1–0.2	
Butorphanol	0.2–0.4	High end dosage for smaller patients. Less analgesia than pure opioids (for mild pain).
Buprenorphine	0.02–0.04	

Alpha₂ agonists		Provide profound sedation and analgesia and greatly spare (≥50%) anesthesia needed. Use alpha₂ agonists *only* in healthy young animals.
Xylazine	0.2–0.4	
Medetomidine	0.01–0.02	
Telazol	2 IM	Good for immobilization of aggressive dogs.
Induction		Administered "to effect" to facilitate unconsciousness and intubation for inhalant anesthesia.
Thiopental	5–10 IV	Apnea is common.
Diazepam-ketamine	1 ml/10 kg IV	Can follow prior tranquilizer administration.
Telazol	0.5–1.0 IV	Can follow prior tranquilizer administration.
Propofol	2–6 IV	Apnea is common if not given slowly.
Etomidate	0.5–2.0 IV	Expensive but sparing of cardiorespiratory function.
Total parenteral anesthesia		Less control over anesthesia depth and duration than inhalation maintenance.

(continues)

Table 10–1 *(Continued)*

Protocol	Dosages (mg/kg)* (IV, IM, SC)*	Comments
Xylazine	0.4	Administration of X/B prior to ketamine minimizes pain of IM ketamine *or* ketamine can be administered IV "to effect."
Butorphanol Ketamine	0.4 10	
Medetomidine	0.01–0.02	Administration of M/B prior to ketamine minimizes pain of IM ketamine *or* ketamine can be administered IV "to effect."
Butorphanol Ketamine	0.4 10	
Butorphanol Diazepam-ketamine	0.4 1 ml/10 kg IV	Diazepam-ketamine is titrated to effect. Not for severely painful procedures.
Premedications as above plus propofol	2–6 (induction) 0.4 CRI (constant rate infusion) or repeat bolus of 0.5–1.0 ml "to effect"	Intubation and oxygen delivery is recommended

Opioid antagonists		
Naloxone	0.001–0.015 IV	May be given IV "to effect" when diluted (1 ml in 9 ml saline). Give matching (IV) dose SC.
Nalmefene	0.001 IV	Longer duration of action than naloxone.
Alpha$_2$ antagonists		
Yohimbine	0.05–0.1 IV	May be given IM but less effective.
Atipamezole	0.07–0.15 IV, IM	
Tolazoline	1–2 IV	May be given IM but less effective.

CRI (mg/kg/min).

*As a general rule, use lower dosage range for IV administration. All routes acceptable unless otherwise specified.

**Use of an opioid with one of these medications is called *neuroleptanalgesia*. The combination has a synergistic effect, providing better sedation than either agent alone.

to diazepam when SC or IM administration is needed, since diazepam causes tissue irritation and has unreliable absorption when given by these routes. Thiopental and diazepam-ketamine are economical and effective induction agents, but repeated bolus administration can contribute to a rough, prolonged recovery and both thiopental and ketamine have specific contraindications (Chapter 2). Thiopental causes prolonged recovery in sighthounds due to an inherent inability to metabolize the drug efficiently; alternatives include diazepam-ketamine and propofol.

Propofol has become a popular drug in veterinary medicine due to its rapid effect, short duration, and lack of cumulative effect, which allows it to be used as repeated boluses or constant rate infusion without significantly increasing recovery time. Even though more expensive than thiopental, propofol's rapid recovery and lack of arrhythmogenic effect make it an excellent alternative agent.

Applying local and regional anesthetic techniques appropriate to the procedure (most conveniently following anesthetic induction) provides preemptive and postoperative analgesia and further decreases anesthetic maintenance requirements.

Dogs are prone to regurgitation and aspiration. Anesthetized patients should be *intubated* to assure a patent and protected airway, especially if fasting status is unknown or time will not permit an adequate fast (emergencies). Dogs are relatively easy to intubate by direct visualization of the larynx, which is aided by adequate anesthetic depth and use of a laryngoscope. Intubation provides a route for oxygen delivery with or without inhalant administration and an effective means for providing ventilatory support. Appropriate tube sizes for dogs cover a wide range from 3.0 to 14.0 mm internal diameter.

An *intravenous catheter* should be placed in a peripheral vein for procedures anticipated to take longer than 30 min and when administration of additional anesthetic agent is likely. The most common sites are the cephalic and lateral saphenous veins. A secure access provides a route for intraoperative fluid and supportive drug administration and for emergency drug administration, should cardiopulmonary arrest occur.

Recovery should occur in a warm quiet area with external heat provided in most cases. Extubation is performed with the cuff deflated when swallowing is noted. When there is evidence of regurgitation or when blood has collected in the pharyngeal region, the oral cavity should be swabbed and the tube removed with the cuff still inflated once swallowing is observed to remove any debris that has settled around the tube within the trachea. Patients with underlying airway compromise (brachycephalic breeds, history of a collapsing trachea) should remain intubated as long as possible and closely observed until recovery is complete. Animals should be observed until vital signs have returned to normal (Chapter 1).

11

Anesthetic Management of Cats

Total parenteral anesthetic protocols seem to be more popular and widely used in cats than dogs for a variety of reasons, including greater resistance to handling and restraint, more difficult venous access, more difficult intubation, and greater effectiveness with less occurrence of side effects associated with dissociative agents. Several protocols are available for short-term injectable anesthesia (Table 11–1). However, for complicated, prolonged procedures and high-risk cats, inhalation maintenance following premedication and induction is more controllable and safer (see Table 11–1).

For tractable patients, neuroleptanalgesic combinations like those used for dogs are effective. Pure opioid agonists have been reported to cause excitement in cats,

Table 11–1   Recommended Dosages and Protocols for Chemical Restraint, Preanesthetic and Induction Protocols, and Total Parenteral Anesthesia for Cats

Protocol	Dosages (mg/kg) (IV, IM, SC)*	Comments
Chemical restraint/ premedication		
Acepromazine or	0.05–0.1	Animals can be aroused during chemical restraint.
Diazepam or	0.2	Benzodiazepines are preferred for high-risk, neonatal, and geriatric patients.
Midazolam	0.1–0.2	
Used with		
Morphine	0.4–1.0	Less analgesia than pure opioids (for mild to moderate pain).
Oxymorphone	0.1–0.2	
Hydromorphone	0.1–0.2	
Butorphanol	0.4	
Induction		
Thiopental	5–10 IV	Administered "to effect" to facilitate unconsciousness and intubation. Apnea is common.
Diazepam-ketamine	1 ml/10 kg IV	Can be used even with prior tranquilizer administration.

Telazol	0.5–1.0 IV	Can be used even with prior tranquilizer administration.
Propofol	2–6 IV	Apnea is common especially with rapid injection.
Etomidate	0.5–2.0 IV	Expensive but sparing of cardiorespiratory function.
Parenteral anesthesia		
Xylazine	0.4	Administration of X/B prior to ketamine will minimize pain of IM ketamine or ketamine can be administered IV "to effect."
Butorphanol	0.4	
Ketamine	10–15	
Medetomidine	0.01–0.02	Administration of M/B prior to ketamine will minimize pain of IM ketamine or ketamine can be administered IV "to effect."
Butorphanol	0.4	
Ketamine	10–15	
Propofol	2–6 (induction) 0.4 constant rate infusion or repeat bolus of 0.25–0.5 "to effect"	Acepromazine or benzodiazepine plus opioid followed by propofol.

Note: Dosages for reversal agents are similar to those listed for dogs (see Table 10–1 or Appendix 1).

*As a general rule, use lower dosage range for IV administration.

but risk of this side effect is minimized with concurrent use of a tranquilizer or when an agonist-antagonist (butorphanol) is used. Adding a low dose of ketamine to the neuroleptanalgesic combination (see Table 11–1) will provide immobilization for less tractable patients to facilitate catheterization and will further decrease induction requirements. While mask induction following premedication is effective in cats, induction quality is improved and intubation facilitated by using a rapid induction method such as thiopental, diazepam-ketamine, telazol, or propofol. The feline respiratory center is more susceptible to the depression associated with thiopental and propofol and transient apnea is common. Some cats will produce excessive respiratory secretions when the dissociative agents are used, which may be counteracted by anticholinergic agent administration.

As a rule, cats tend to resent and resist restraint more than dogs. Various devices, such as cat bags and feline muzzles, often are necessary to ensure the safety of personnel and the animal. Always close the doors to avoid escape when working with cats. Most cats can be restrained adequately with scruffing and stretching (holding the skin behind the neck with one hand and the rear limbs with the other and applying gentle tension) for injection of premedication. For resistant animals, adding ketamine or telazol in low dosage to the premedication protocol improves the quality of the catheterization/induction sequence. Many of the local and regional techniques, such as epidural and local nerve blocks, are effective and feasible in cats to provide preemptive and postoperative analgesia (Chapter 3).

When indicated (high-risk animal, repeat injections, prolonged procedures), an IV catheter should be inserted. Cats seem to resist the necessary restraint as much as the actual catheter placement so premedication usually is required. Sites include the cephalic, medial saphenous, and femoral veins. Laying the animal in lateral recumbency for placement in the medial saphenous vein seems to be less stressful for some anxious, aggressive patients.

Feline intubation is more challenging than in dogs. While visualization usually is good, the feline larynx is reactive and prone to laryngospasm, which makes intubation more difficult and increases the risk of trauma. Patience is essential, and the process is facilitated by application of 0.1 ml of 2% lidocaine dropped from a syringe to desensitize the area. Commercial human spray preparations containing benzocaine (e.g., Cetacaine™) should be avoided because of reports of methemoglobinemia associated with its use. Once visualized and desensitized, using a guide tube (canine polyethylene urinary catheter) will help to stiffen the ET tube and gain access between the arytenoid cartilages and into the trachea so that the tube may be passed, rotating slightly if needed, to allow the bevel to pass into the trachea. Stiffer stylets are available, but the risk of trauma is greater if care is not taken to maintain the stylet point inside the ET tube. The tube is secured around the back of the neck with tie gauze.

While a standard rebreathing circle can be used effectively in cats, a pediatric circle or nonrebreathing system is more appropriate for their size. The latter will minimize resistance to breathing but is more likely to contribute to intraoperative hypothermia. If a rebreathing circuit is used, ventilatory support becomes even more important (due to added resistance to breathing), especially during prolonged procedures.

Cats are more challenging to monitor. The smaller tidal volume makes movement of the rebreathing bag more difficult to observe. Esophageal stethoscopes are helpful forausculting both respiration and heart sounds. Respiratory monitors and capnometers usually are effective but add to dead space. Pulse quality is more difficult to assess; the best site for pulse palpation is the femoral artery, which may not always be accessible. The dorsal pedal artery can be palpated in some cats; clipping the area over this artery is beneficial. Pulse oximeters and oscillometric blood pressure monitors may fail to work consistently, due to the small vessel size. The Doppler apparatus is effective when applied to either a forelimb or hindlimb but takes time and experience to apply efficiently. The feline lead II electrocardiogram is small and sometimes difficult to assess.

Recovery usually is rapid in cats following inhalation anesthesia, unless severe hypothermia has developed. Providing a warm environment and thermal support facilitate recovery. Close attention to body temperature is important, as cats seem prone to hyperthermia as body activity increases during recovery, seemingly independent of the protocol used. As a general rule, once the body temperature reaches 99°F, thermal support should be removed. Cats with elevated temperature (>104°F) benefit from the application of alcohol to the pads and a fan to dissipate heat; animals act seemingly normal during this period of increased temperature; thermoregulation returns to normal usually within 24 hr.

12

Anesthetic Management of Birds

Birds frequently require general anesthesia for a veterinarian to perform procedures normally accomplished with physical restraint in most other species as well as complicated and invasive procedures. General anesthesia is challenging in birds due to less familiarity with avian anatomy, greater resistance to restraint, lower margin of safety for injectable agents, less experience with catheterization and intubation techniques, more difficulty in monitoring, and currently, limited information on effective analgesic agents.

Capture and restraint should be performed in a quiet and safe environment and done quickly to minimize the stress of chasing. Passeriformes may be restrained with the bird cradled in the palm of the hand and the head gently restrained between the index and middle fingers. For the larger Psittaciformes, a two-hand technique is required (Figure 12–1). Head restraint is vital to avoid bites to the handler and accomplished by creating a ring around the bird's neck with one hand and applying gentle pressure against the base of the skull and lower mandible. The other hand is placed around the legs to gently support the body. A towel can be used to protect the hand near the head. It is essential to not restrict thoracic movement or compromise the airway. Restraint techniques for adult ratites cannot be described in the confines of this reference book; for information, readers are referred to the recommended reading list.

Anesthetic induction and maintenance with isoflurane is the protocol of choice for pet birds and raptors. Sevoflurane also appears to be effective and currently is gaining popularity. Dosages for some injectable protocols are available and listed in Table 12–1; however, these agents usually fail to produce stable and safe levels of anesthesia and should not be used unless gas anesthesia is unavailable. Larger birds, such as ratites, will require an injectable premedication and induction protocol (see Table 12–1) because mask induction is prolonged and dangerous except in debilitated patients.

Intubation is relatively easy to perform in avian species as the glottis is readily apparent at the base of the tongue when the beak is opened. Psittaciformes have a fleshy tongue, which must be pulled forward carefully to expose the glottis. Birds >350 grams can be intubated

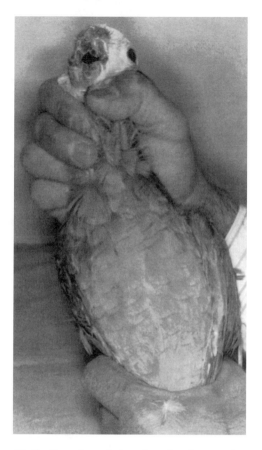

Figure 12–1 Restraint technique for Psittaciformes, demonstrating hand positioning. (Reprinted with permission from TG Curro, Anesthesia of pet birds, in: *Seminars in Avian and Exotic Pet Medicine: Anesthesia and Analgesia*, AM Fudge, ed., 1998;7(1):12.)

Table 12–1 Reported Dosages for Injectable Anesthetic Agents in Pet Birds, Raptors, and Ratites (Injectable protocols are not recommended in birds unless inhalant anesthesia is unavailable.)

Drug Combination	Dosage (mg/kg)*
*Pet birds***	
Ketamine-xylazine	10–50/1.0–10
Ketamine-diazepam	10–50/0.5–2.0
Ketamine-midazolam	10–40/0.5–1.5
Ketamine-acepromazine	10–25/0.5–1.0
Telazol (tiletamine-zolazepam)	7.7–26.0
Yohimbine	1.0
Analgesic options	
Butorphanol	1–4 IV, SC, IM
Flunixin	1–10 IM (not critically evaluated)
Aspirin	5 gr/250 ml drinking water (not critically evaluated)
Raptors†	
Buteo Hawks	
350 g	0.04–0.08 ml
650–1500 g	0.08–0.15 ml
900–1700 g	0.1–0.3 ml
Accipiter Hawks	
100–250 g	0.04–0.06 ml
250–500 g	0.08–0.1 ml
600–1200 g	0.05–0.07 ml

(continues)

Table 12-1 *(Continued)*

Drug Combination	Dosage (mg/kg)*
Eagles	
3–5 kg	0.1–0.2 ml
Falcons	
90–250 g	0.03–0.06 ml
500–950 g	0.07–0.2 ml
950–1500 g	0.12–0.3 ml
Owls	
60–130 g	0.03–0.05
150–350 g	0.05–0.1
700–2500 g	0.1–0.25 (not recommended for surgery on great horned or snowy owls)
Osprey	0.12–0.2 ml
Turkey vulture	0.15–0.2 ml
Ratites	
Xylazine	0.2–2.2 IM
Detomidine	1.5 IM
Medetomidine	0.1 IM
Butorphanol	0.05–0.5 IV, IM
Diazepam	0.1–0.3 IV
	0.22–1.0 IM
Midazolam	0.15 IM
Ketamine-xylazine	2.2 IV/0.25 IV
	2.2–3.3 IV/2.2 IM
Carfentanil-xylazine	0.03 IV/0.5 IM

(continues)

Table 12–1 (Continued)

Drug Combination	Dosage (mg/kg)*
Ketamine-diazepam	5.0/0.25 IV (mixed) 2.2–3.3 IV/0.22–0.5 IM (ketamine given 15–30 min after diazepam)
Telazol	2–10 IM; 1–3 IV
Antagonists:	
Naloxone	2 mg IV (total dose administered to adult ostriches)
Yohimbine	12.5 mg IV (total dose administered to adult ostriches)
Atipamezole	5–20 mg IV (total dose administered to adult ostriches)
Naltrexone	300 mg IV (total dose administered to adult ostriches)

*Dosages are for intramuscular administration in the pectoral muscles unless otherwise indicated.

**Lower dosage range is for larger birds (>250 g) and sedation in smaller birds; higher dosage range is for smaller birds (<250 g) and for a "surgical plane" of anesthesia in larger birds.

†Dosage in mls of a mixture of 1 ml ketamine (100 mg/ml) and xylazine (20 mg/ml). Low-end range represents minimal effective dose, high-end range represents surgical anesthesia. As with pet birds, injectable anesthesia is not recommended for raptors. A dosage range for the xylazine-ketamine mixture (100 mg/20 mg) has been published and dosages in ml are summarized. For details on anesthetic management of raptors and other species, see PT Redig, Recommendations for anesthesia in raptors with comments on trumpeter swans, in: *Seminars in Avian and Exotic Pet Medicine: Anesthesia and Analgesia,* AM Fudge, ed., 1998;7(1):22–29.

with a cuffed tube (smallest: 3.0–5.0 mm ID). Larger raptors may require slightly larger tubes, and the adult ratite trachea accommodates tube sizes up to 18 mm ID. Birds 100–350 g require uncuffed tubes (2.0–3.0 mm ID), Cole tubes (uncuffed tubes with a tapered end), or large gauge IV catheters (14–18 ga). Birds smaller than 100 g are best maintained by mask with the head gently extended because there is an increased likelihood of tube occlusion and significant impedance to air movement associated with the small diameter catheters required in this size bird. Endotracheal tubes with a side opening near the bevel (Murphy tubes) help minimize the risk of mucus occlusion. Once in place, the tube is effectively secured with a thin piece of tape around the tube, which then is encircled around the closed beak.

For cases with airway obstruction or to perform procedures in the oral cavity, inhalant anesthesia can be delivered into the air sacs. Percutaneous catheters (14–18 ga; 2–3 cm) may be placed in the caudal thoracic or abdominal air sacs using sterile technique. A small skin incision is required to expose the air sac membrane. The catheter is inserted and the skin secured around the catheter; the catheter is connected to an endotracheal tube adaptor for delivery of the anesthetic agent. The approximate site of entry is at the last intercostal space. Apnea is common when this technique is used, making monitoring of cardiovascular parameters critical.

For prolonged procedures or debilitated patients and when significant hemorrhage is anticipated, intraoperative fluids should be administered. Intravenous access is possible in birds weighing ≥250 grams; sites include the jugular, cutaneous ulnar, and medial metatarsal veins. When fluid administration is essential and IV access unsuccessful, the intraosseous route also is effective. Sites of entry include the distal ulna and the proximal tibiotarsus (Figure 12–2). Spinal or hypodermic needles are used, depending on the size of the bird; the former minimizes the risk of needle occlusion by a bone core during placement. Once placed, the needle is capped and secured as for an IV catheter. Subcutaneous fluid administration sites include the propatagium (wing web), intrascapular, and inguinal regions. Dextrose-containing fluids (LRS or Normosol with 2.5–5.0% dextrose, half strength LRS, or saline with 2.5% dextrose) are recommended. Fluids administered SC should contain ≤2.5% dextrose.

Sensitivity to anesthesia is variable among avian species and individual birds can develop complications rapidly; therefore, monitoring heart and respiratory rates is essential. Effective aids to anesthetic monitoring include direct or esophageal auscultation, a lead II electrocardiogram (Figure 12–3), and respiratory (apnea) monitor; the last may not function effectively in very small patients, adds dead space to the breathing circuit, and usually is ineffective during mask delivery. Placement of ECG leads include the skin of the propatagium

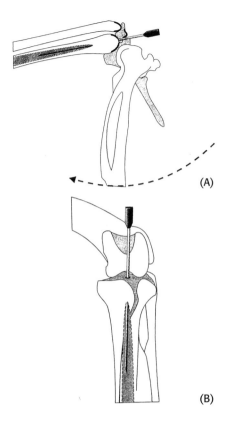

Figure 12–2 Sites for intraosseous catheterization of birds for intraoperative fluid administration: (A) site for placing spinal or hypodermic needle via the distal ulna; (B) site for placing spinal or hypodermic needle via the proximal tibiotarsus. (Reprinted with permission from DJ Harris, Therapeutic avian techniques, in: *Seminars in Avian and Exotic Pet Medicine: Clinical Techniques*, AM Fudge, ed., 1997;6(2):61.)

(LA and RA) and the skin of the stifle (LL). Alligator clips should be padded with alcohol-soaked gauze to avoid skin damage or, alternatively and effective, snap-on sticky ECG pads can be applied. Heart rates should remain between 200 and 400 beats/min depending on the size of the bird (less for large ratites: 60–120 beats/min). During surgical anesthesia, birds should be relaxed and unresponsive to painful stimulation; corneal and pedal reflexes are slow and the palpebral reflex is lost. Respiration should be slow, regular, and deep, with rates usually ranging from 12–30 breaths/min. Temperature should be monitored, especially during long procedures, to avoid development of hypothermia. External heat sources should be provided; maintaining a body temperature of 101–103°F is recommended.

Recovery usually occurs within 5–15 min after inhalant delivery is discontinued and should occur in a warm, quiet, and dimly lit environment. Birds should be wrapped loosely in a towel and gently restrained until extubated and able to stand. For prolonged recovery, birds may be left in a padded enclosure with close observation, once extubated. For extubation, the oral cavity should be checked for regurgitation or excessive secretions and swabbed if needed. Extubation should be performed when the bird resists its presence. Information on analgesic agent dosages for birds is limited but should be considered for painful invasive procedures and administered either intraoperatively or just prior to recovery. Dosages for butorphanol have been reported

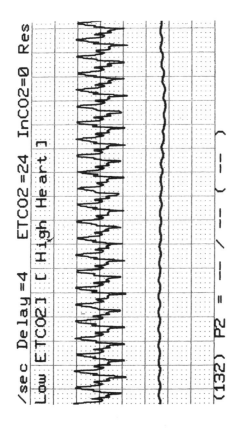

Figure 12-3 Normal ECG (with a simultaneous arterial pressure wave) from a 260 g Hispaniolan Amazon parrot. Heart rate was about 400 beats/min.

for pet birds and probably can be extrapolated to raptors. Flunixin meglumate and aspirin also have been recommended but not critically evaluated. Dosages are listed in Table 12–1. Birds should be offered food and water when able to perch.

13

Anesthetic Management of Small Mammals

This chapter primarily addresses anesthetic management of rabbits and ferrets with additional comments on management and analgesic options for other small mammals.

Ferrets

Ferrets are effectively restrained (and often resent it less) by techniques established for use in cats; namely, "scruffing" the skin of the neck and gently stretching the animal by grasping the rear limbs. Premedication is recommended in all but extremely debilitated animals; protocols are listed in Table 13–1. Most ferrets can be catheterized for IV induction following a neuroleptanalgesic combination, although healthy, uncooperative patients will benefit from the addition of ketamine to the preanesthetic protocol. Induction may be accomplished by inhalant anesthetic, preferably isoflurane, delivered by mask, or with an IV protocol such as thiopental, diazepam-ketamine, or propofol; IV induction will provide more reliable access and increased duration of time for intubation.

Sites for intravenous catheterization in ferrets include the cephalic, lateral saphenous, and (last) the jugular veins. Skin is tough, so making an "introduction hole" through the skin over the vein with a hypodermic needle to facilitate entry of the catheter (22 or 24 ga) is beneficial. Placing a tourniquet above the site will help maximally raise the vessel, which is very difficult to visualize due to its small size and the usual presence of a large amount of SC fat. Catheterization is recommended for prolonged procedures and high-risk patients to provide access for administration of intraoperative fluids and anticipated supportive measures.

Intubation is relatively easy in ferrets. Visualization is similar to cats and the ferret larynx usually will accommodate a 2.5–3.0 mm ID tube. The larynx is less reactive than cats, making local anesthetic desensitization unnecessary; visualization is facilitated by a laryngoscope. The tube should be secured around the back of the head with tie gauze as it is in cats.

Table 13–1 Dosages of Premedication Protocols and Induction Agents for Ferrets and Rabbits

Protocol	Dosage (mg/kg)	Comments
Ferrets		
Premedication/ chemical restraint		
Atropine	0.05 SC, IV, IM	Routine use not recommended.
Glycopyrrolate	0.01 SC, IV, IM	Routine use not recommended.
Acepromazine/ butorphanol	0.1/0.4 SC	Avoid acepromazine in debilitated patients. Add ketamine (5–10 mg/kg IM) to provide immobilization to facilitate catheterization, induction, and minor procedures.
Midazolam/ butorphanol	0.2–0.4/0.4 SC	Good for debilitated patients. Diazepam (0.2–2.0 mg/kg) may be used in place of midazolam but is less well absorbed and causes pain on injection. Add ketamine (5–10 mg/kg IM) to provide immobilization to facilitate catheterization, induction, and minor procedures.

(continues)

Table 13–1   *(Continued)*

Protocol	Dosage (mg/kg)	Comments
Xylazine	0.5–1.0 SC	For healthy patients only. Not recommended as a premedication for inhalant anesthetic maintenance.
Medetomidine	0.08 SC	For healthy patients only. Not recommended as a premedication for inhalant anesthetic maintenance.
Telazol	6–12 IM	Recovery may be prolonged (>4 hr). Reported side effects include sneezing and paddling during induction and recovery. Facilitates minor noninvasive procedures.
*Induction**		
Thiopental	8–12 IV	Give slowly "to effect."
Ketamine plus diazepam or midazolam	0.1 ml/kg IV	Drug mixture is made by combining *equal volumes* of ketamine and benzodiazepine. Give "to effect."
Propofol	2–5 IV	Give slowly "to effect."
*Injectable mixtures***		
Acepromazine/ ketamine	0.2–0.3/20–30 IM	

Xylazine/ketamine	2.0/25 IM	Anecdotal reports of death in apparently normal animals have been associated with xylazine-ketamine.
Acepromazine/ xylazine/ ketamine	0.05/1–2/20–30 IM	
Medetomidine/ butorphanol/ ketamine	0.08/0.1/10 IM	Giving other agents SC prior to IM ketamine will help minimize the pain of IM injection.
Rabbits†		
Premedication/ chemical restraint		
Atropine	0.04–0.5 SC, IV, IM	Routine use not recommended.
Glycopyrrolate	0.01 SC, IV, IM	Routine use not recommended.
Acepromazine/ buprenorphine/ ketamine	0.1 SC/0.04 SC/ 5–10 IM	Give ketamine 10–15 minutes after other agents or give all IM; ketamine may not be necessary in tractable patients. Facilitates catheterization, induction, and minor noninvasive procedures.

(continues)

Table 13–1 (Continued)

Protocol	Dosage (mg/kg)	Comments
Midazolam or diazepam/ butorphanol/ ketamine	0.2 SC (IM for diazepam)/0.4 SC/5–10 IM	Midazolam provides more reliable absorption and less pain on injection. Ketamine may not be needed for tractable or depressed patients. Good alternative for debilitated patients. Facilitates catheterization, induction, and minor noninvasive procedures.
Telazol	5–11 IM	Facilitates catheterization, induction, and minor noninvasive procedures. Recoveries may be prolonged. Nephrotoxicity has been reported but unlikely at these doses.
*Induction**		
Diazepam/ketamine	1 ml/5–10 kg IV	A 1:1 (volume) mixture given to effect.
Propofol	4–10 IV	Administer *slowly* to avoid apnea.
*Injectable mixtures***		
Xylazine/ketamine	5/35	For healthy animals *only*. Provides ≤ 30 minutes of surgical anesthesia. Response is variable and ineffective in some patients.

Profound hypoxemia is reported with this combination; supplemental oxygen is recommended.

*Mask induction is effective in ferrets and rabbits following premedication and recommended in debilitated patients. Mask induction is particularly appropriate in rabbits because maintenance of anesthesia via mask is very common due to difficult intubation. Rapid acting IV agents provide superior relaxation and visualization of the larynx and more time to successfully complete intubation. Telazol and combinations including ketamine may allow intubation without masking or additional injectable agents.

**Injectable combinations provide short duration anesthesia for minor procedures and the dosages listed are not those recommended for administration prior to inhalant maintenance. Patients should be closely monitored when combinations that include alpha$_2$ agonists are used and alpha$_2$ agonist-containing combinations are not recommended prior to inhalant maintenance.

†Effectiveness of intranasal administration of several anesthetic protocols has been reported in rabbits and provides an alternative route for premedication administration. Effective (and relatively safe) protocols (mg/kg) include xylazine (3)/ketamine (10); midazolam (2); ketamine (25); midazolam (1)/ketamine (25); telazol (10). Onset time was within 3 min. None of the protocols provided consistent evidence of adequate anesthesia for invasive procedures.

Effective monitoring devices include an esophageal stethoscope, ECG, respiratory monitor, capnometer, and pulse oximeter.

Ferrets lose body heat rapidly, and external heat must be provided. Recovery should occur in a warm, quiet environment; an incubator is ideal, especially when significant hypothermia has developed, which is common during abdominal procedures. Options for postoperative analgesia are listed in Table 13–2.

Rabbits

Rabbits are easily stressed by handling, which can have a negative impact on the anesthetic period. When frightened, they may hold deceptively still then struggle to escape, which can predispose them to traumatic fractures of the vertebral column (due to the massive rear limb muscles and low-density skeletal system) or exhibit a rapid ventilatory rate (200 breaths/min), which might be misinterpreted as a respiratory abnormality. *Safe restraint* is essential to avoid injury, performed by gently grasping the skin of the neck and supporting the body on the forearm or a nonslip table. Loosely wrapping the rabbit in a towel or restraint bag also helps minimize injury. The immobility reflex ("hypnosis") has been described for rabbits and can facilitate minor procedures, such as physical examination and blood collection. Briefly, the rabbit is placed in dorsal recumbency and gentle traction applied to the neck while rubbing

Table 13–2 Dosages of Selected Analgesic Agents for a Variety of Small Mammal Species

Drug	Ferret	Rabbit	Rat, Hamster, Gerbil	Guinea Pig, Chinchilla	Mouse
Opioids					
Buprenorphine	0.01–0.03/ 8–12 IV, SC	0.01–0.05/ 8–12 SC	0.01–0.05/ 8–12 SC, IV / 0.05/ 8–12 SC	0.1–0.25/ 8–12 PO	0.05–0.1/ 12 SC
Butorphanol	0.4/4–6 SC	0.1–0.5/ 2–4 SC	2.0/4 SC	1.0–2.0/4 SC	1.0–5.0/SC
Morphine	0.5–5.0/ 6 SC	2.0–5.0/ 2–4 SC	2.0–5.0/ 2–4 SC	2.0–5.0/ 2–4 SC	2.0–5.0/ 2–4 SC
NSAIDs					
Aspirin	200/* PO	100/* PO	100/* PO	87/* PO	120/* PO
Carprofen**	2.0–4.0/ 24 SC	1.5/12 PO	5.0/24 SC	NA	5.0/* SC
Flunixin meglumate	0.5–2.0/ 12–24 SC	1.1/12 SC	2.5/12 SC	1–2/* SC	2.5/12 SC

(continues)

Table 13–2 (Continued)

Drug	Ferret	Rabbit	Rat, Hamster, Gerbil	Guinea Pig, Chinchilla	Mouse
Ketoprofen	NA	3.0/* IM, SC	5.0/* SC	NA	NA

Note: Numbers represent dosage in mg/kg /interval (in hr) for each species category. Considerable individual variation in response exists in these species and frequent assessment of efficacy is critical.

*Reliable data regarding dosage interval is unavailable. Conservative dosing at 12–24 hr interval is recommended. In general, NSAIDs should not be used for more than 1–3 days, due to the potential adverse side effects and paucity of information regarding safety in these species.

**Carprofen currently is not available in the injectable form in the United States.

Routes of administration:

IV = intravenous

SC = subcutaneous

IM = intramuscular

PO = oral

NA = not available

Dosages are adapted from PA Flecknell, Analgesia in small mammals, in: *Seminars in Avian and Exotic Pet Medicine: Anesthesia and Analgesia,* AM Fudge, ed., 1998;7(1):41–47. (Dosages for hamsters, gerbils, and chinchillas are based on extrapolation from other species and initial doses should utilize the lower dosage range.)

the abdomen. The hypnotized rabbit usually stays still for a short period of time, unless aroused by loud noises or rough handling.

Premedication usually is required to facilitate smooth induction of anesthesia, and protocols are listed in Table 13–1. Most of the agents may be administered subcutaneously (over the skin of the back), and this is preferred, due to occasional occurrence of lameness and tissue necrosis associated with IM administration. Dissociative agents should be administered IM, and the most common sites include the anterior and posterior thigh. A significant percentage of rabbits (30–50%) possess atropinesterase, which results in rapid metabolism and abbreviated effective duration of atropine. Because of this, a wide range of dosages has been recommended in the literature; however, routine use is unnecessary and anticholinergic agent administration in rabbits is best reserved for treatment of intraoperative bradycardia (HR <70–80/min or an abrupt, marked decrease [≥20%] in HR). Dosages for atropine and glycopyrrolate are listed in Table 13–1.

Intravenous catheterization following premedication usually is possible in rabbits over 2 kg and recommended for prolonged procedures, debilitated patients, and to facilitate IV induction of anesthesia. Sites include the cephalic, lateral saphenous, and marginal ear veins, using a 22–24 ga catheter. The ear vein is particularly fragile and more difficult to catheterize than the other two sites.

Mask induction, preferably with isoflurane, is an effective method when the rabbit is adequately restrained and sedated; and it is particularly applicable when intubation is not planned. For prolonged procedures, intubation is recommended; and a rapid-acting induction agent, such as diazepam-ketamine, propofol, or thiopental, will facilitate the process. Intranasal administration of anesthetic agents for sedation or to induce anesthesia also has been reported for rabbits and may provide an alternative route for some agents in specific individuals (Table 13–1).

Rabbits are difficult to intubate and it takes practice and anatomical knowledge to master the technique. The endotracheal tube size for rabbits ranges 2.0–4.0 mm ID. The oral cavity is small but long, with limited ability for the animal to open its mouth. The tongue tends to obscure the larynx. The epiglottis is long and pliable, often remaining dorsal to the soft palate. The pharynx is located at a right angle to the larynx, and the larynx is susceptible to laryngospasm and trauma.

Adequate anesthetic depth is essential to facilitate atraumatic intubation, and several methods and animal positions (with sternal recumbency being most common) have been described. The head and neck should be kept in full extension; a length of roll gauze placed behind the upper incisors will help hold the mouth open; and retraction of the tongue lateral to the lower incisors will minimize risk of laceration during the procedure. Techniques include *blind* (passing the tube to the point of maximum intensity of breath sounds either with the ear or with stethoscope earpieces attached to the end of the tube, then passing the tube during inspiration when the larynx is maximally abducted) and *direct visualization* (with a small lighted laryngoscope or otoscope to guide the tube into place). Use of an introductory tube, such as a small urinary catheter, placed visually into the larynx may facilitate the process. A drop of 1% or 2% lidocaine on the glottis will help minimize laryngospasm. Evidence of proper placement includes a cough reflex with passage and those signs previously noted in Chapter 9. Roll gauze tied around the tube and around the back of the head will secure the tube in place.

Once induction is complete, epidural administration of local anesthetic agents, with or without an opioid, is effective and relatively easy to perform in rabbits to provide preemptive analgesia for procedures involving the abdomen and hind limbs. Dosages and technique are similar to those described for dogs and cats (Chapter 3).

Monitoring tools, to enhance observation of breathing rate (>15 breaths/min) and pattern and auscultation/palpation of pulse rate (auricular, femoral, or dorsal pedal), include the ECG and, in larger rabbits, noninvasive blood pressure monitors placed over a peripheral artery. Pulse oximetry has limited use (due to frequent use of a mask for maintenance and limited exposure of the tongue for probe placement), but may work on the ear in light-skinned rabbits. Respiratory

devices and the esophageal stethoscope require intubation and, so, often are not applicable. Respiratory dysfunction probably is the most common anesthetic
complication in rabbits and close observation of the
breathing rate and pattern is essential. A sudden change
in these parameters should prompt assessment of ET
tube patency (if in place) or the oropharynx for excessive secretions (if a mask is used), and anesthetic delivery
should be decreased or stopped. Reflexes used to assess
anesthetic depth include the pinna ("ear pinch") and
pedal reflexes with the former considered to be most
reliable. The palpebral reflex has been reported to be
unreliable in rabbits; loss of the corneal reflex, as in
other species, indicates excessive anesthetic depth.

Monitoring should continue into the recovery
period, until the animal is extubated and vital signs are
stable, and should proceed in a warm environment (with
incubator or heat lamp support) until the animal's temperature returns to normal (Chapter 1). Analgesic agent
dosages have been reported (see Table 13–2) and should
be applied to rabbits subjected to painful procedures to
help minimize stress and suffering.

Other Small Mammals

A variety of "pocket pets" may be presented with the need
for general anesthesia. Some general statements regarding management in clinical situations can be made:

1. For small mammals, anesthetic management is best accomplished by mask or chamber induction (depending on tractability) with isoflurane or sevoflurane. Designing a mask to work effectively may require some innovative modification of standard feline or canine masks or syringe cases. Intubation may be attempted if the necessary tube sizes and adjunct equipment are available.

2. When dealing with species for which anesthetic dosage and technique information is limited, efforts to minimize anesthesia time is essential.

3. Established monitoring tools often are effective; it is always worthwhile to apply available equipment, especially during prolonged procedures.

4. Venous access is not always possible with small mammals, but when fluid therapy is indicated, alternative routes, including SC and intraosseous, should be considered.

5. Analgesic therapy should be considered for any animal undergoing a painful procedure; when specific dosages are not readily available, extrapolation or scrutiny of the literature may provide safe, effective guidelines. Table 13–2 provides dosages of analgesic agents in a variety of small mammal species.

14

Anesthetic Management of Reptiles

A variety of reptilian species may be presented with the need for chemical restraint and general anesthesia, and this represents a unique challenge, including limited sites for parenteral agent injection and IV access, a major tendency to become apneic during anesthesia (which often prevents use of mask induction), difficulty in cardiac auscultation, and limited usefulness of available monitoring tools.

Restraint techniques are relatively simple for most reptiles but may become more challenging in infrequently encountered aggressive patients. Lizards are restrained by enclosing in the hand if small or securing on a flat surface then applying gentle pressure to the neck and caudal body. For snakes, a hand should secure the head and the remainder of the body supported with the other hand or on a flat surface. Turtles require minimal restraint but present a unique problem in that the head usually is inaccessible for physical examination. To view the head, applying a gentle pinch to a front limb usually will cause it to emerge from the shell. Two preanesthetic considerations are important for reptiles. Allow at least 24 hr of hospitalization prior to anesthesia for acclimation. The optimal temperature for most species is 86–88°F. Second, an accurate weight is important to calculate dosages for premedication, which is necessary for induction in most reptile patients. Fasting in reptiles generally is not recommended; the exception is snakes, for which a large meal ingested just prior to anesthesia could impede cardiovascular function; therefore, a 24-hr (minimum) fast is recommended.

Various sites for blood collection have been reported—lizards (toenail, ventral tail vein); snakes (ventral tail vein, heart, palatine vein); turtles (toenail, brachial plexus)—and may be required for the workup of complicated cases.

Induction and intubation for maintenance with inhalant anesthesia (preferably isoflurane) is facilitated by IM administration of ketamine. Dosages for ketamine and other adjunct drugs are listed in Table 14–1. None of the agents listed provides adequate analgesia alone and inhalant supplementation is necessary for painful procedures. Because many species of reptiles can convert to anaerobic metabolism and become apneic, mask induction is prolonged without the benefit of an injectable agent. Like birds, reptiles have a renal portal system and the caudal half of the body should be avoided for IM drug administration. Sites for IM injection include the front legs (lizards, chelonians) and the paravertebral muscles (lizards, snakes). A nonrebreathing system for inhalant delivery is recommended for reptiles weighing <5 kg.

Intubation is important in anesthetic management of reptiles to provide ventilatory support during the anesthetic period and maintain an adequate depth of anesthesia. Intubation is relatively easy to perform and can be accomplished in some awake reptiles, including snakes and some iguanas. The glottis is located rostrally and hence easy to view. However, the glottis is closed at rest and patience is required to wait for an inspiration to allow passage of the tube. The tube may be passed through the closed glottis *if extreme care is taken* and may be facilitated by passage of a soft stylet (urinary catheter) to guide the entry of the endotracheal tube. Tube sizes for reptiles range from 2.0–4.0 mm ID, but smaller patients may require other options, such as IV catheters. Short tubes should be used in turtles, due to their relatively short trachea. Chelonians have complete tracheal rings, making them susceptible to mucosal damage due to an overinflated cuff; snakes and lizards have incomplete tracheal rings. When a cuffed tube is used in any reptile, care should be taken to *not* overinflate the cuff.

Table 14–1 Dosages for Injectable Anesthetic Agents in Reptiles

Agent	Dosage (mg/kg)*	Comments
Atropine	0.01–0.04	Routine use is not recommended.
Glycopyrrolate	0.01	Routine use is not recommended.
Tranquilizers/alpha$_2$ agonists/antagonists		Dosage and efficacy information is limited.
Acepromazine	0.1–0.5	
Diazepam	0.2–1.0	
Midazolam	0.2–2.0	
Xylazine	0.1–1.25	
Medetomidine	0.1–0.15	
Atipamezole	0.5–0.75	
Neuroleptanalgesia		
Butorphanol/midazolam	0.4/2.0	
Dissociative agents		
Ketamine		Ketamine is the most common anesthetic adjunct utilized.
Lizards	30–50	
Snakes	20–40	

Turtles	30	
Telazol	5–10	May contribute significantly to a prolonged recovery.
Other agents		
Propofol		
Lizards	10 IO	
Snakes	10 IV, IC	
Turtles	5–10 IV	
Analgesic agents		
Butorphanol	0.4 IM, IV, SC	
Buprenorphine	0.01	
Carprofen	2.0–4.0 PO once every 1–3 days	
Flunixin	0.1–0.5 IM once daily (maximum of 3 days)	

IO = intraosseous

IC = intracardiac

*Administration is IM unless otherwise noted.

Intraoperative fluid administration is not routine, unless the procedure is prolonged or the animal debilitated. Intravenous access is a daunting task in reptiles, requiring a cutdown in most cases. The exception is large snakes, in which the palatine vein can be easily visualized and catheterized with a 24 ga catheter following induction and intubation. When needed, the intraosseous route is feasible. Intraosseous catheter sites in lizards include the humerus and tibia. In chelonians, the jugular vein may be catheterized in some patients (sometimes without a cutdown); the long bones lack a distinct medullary canal, limiting IO sites to the bridge between the plastron (bottom of shell) and carapace (top of shell), which may be difficult to enter without penetrating the coelomic cavity.

Ventilatory support at a rate of 6–12 breaths/min should be provided for all reptiles, regardless of the individual's spontaneous rate, to help maintain an adequate plane of anesthesia.

Monitoring anesthetized reptiles is the ultimate challenge. Apnea is common, making respiratory monitoring undependable. Heart sounds are extremely difficult to auscultate, and peripheral pulses rarely are palpable. Useful tools include the ECG (Figure 14–1) and the Doppler blood flow probe (apparatus), which provides an audible signal of cardiac function. The crystal is placed over the heart in snakes and lizards and at the thoracic inlet in chelonians. Reptiles relax in a cranial to caudal direction during anesthesia, and function returns in the opposite direction during recovery. The righting reflex is lost first, followed by the tail- and toe-pinch when a surgical plane of anesthesia is reached. While considerable variation exists, loss of the vent reflex (tail or toe movement when the vent is squeezed), the corneal reflex, and tongue withdrawal all may indicate excessive depth of anesthesia, which should prompt critical patient assessment.

Recovery from inhalation anesthesia often is prolonged in reptiles compared to mammals, commonly taking 1 hr or more, especially following prolonged procedures. Animals should recover in a quiet environment, ideally with the ambient temperature near the species' optimal range. Ventilatory support should be continued to aid in elimination of the anesthetic agent; animals that do not resume spontaneous ventilation within 15 min of discontinuation of anesthetic delivery may benefit from doxapram (5 mg/kg IM). Voluntary movement and increased muscle tone usually are the first signs to indicate extubation, which should be delayed, if possible, until the righting reflex returns. While information is limited, analgesia should be provided for painful procedures. Suggested agents and dosages are listed in Table 14–1.

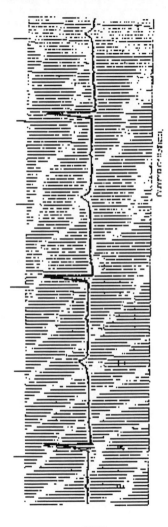

Figure 14–1 Lead II electrocardiogram from an iguana during isoflurane anesthesia. Leads were placed on the forelimbs and left rear limb.

15

Anesthetic Management of Horses

Horses are an anesthetic challenge due to their size, wide range of temperaments, tendency to react explosively to fear and stress, increased risk of trauma associated with induction and recovery (which can both be rough and unpredictable), susceptibility to hypotension, and increased risk for development of postoperative myopathy and neuropathy following inhalant anesthesia. Most short procedures (<60 min) in horses are performed with total parenteral anesthesia, using the same agents that provide induction for inhalant anesthesia; recommended protocols are listed in Table 15–1.

Fasting is controversial in horses. Horses cannot vomit, so risk of regurgitation and aspiration is negligible; however, a minimum of 6 hr is recommended. It is

Table 15–1   Protocols for Chemical Restraint, Induction of Anesthesia, and Injectable Anesthesia in Horses

Agent/Protocol	Dosages (mg/kg)	Comments
Adults		
Chemical restraint		
Acepromazine	0.02–0.06	May be combined with alpha$_2$ agonist or opioid.
Xylazine	0.2–1.0	May be combined with acepromazine or opioid.
Detomidine	0.01–0.04	May be combined with acepromazine or opioid.
Butorphanol	0.02–0.04	Usually combined with alpha$_2$ agonist.
Morphine	0.05	Do not use alone due to likelihood of excitement; usually combined with alpha$_2$ agonist.
Induction/short-term anesthesia		
Xylazine/ketamine	1.1*/2.2 IV	Give xylazine first and proceed in 5 min or when sedation appears adequate. For unruly animals, xylazine may be administered IM (2.2 mg/kg) and may require additional IV xylazine (0.2–0.4 mg/kg) prior to ketamine administration. Adjunct drugs to improve

		sedation prior to ketamine include acepromazine (0.02 mg/kg IV or IM) or butorphanol (0.02–0.04 mg/kg IV).
Xylazine/ diazepam/ ketamine	0.5–1.1/0.05–0.1/2.2	Good for debilitated patients and neonates; xylazine administration should precede induction and dose is based on patient alertness. Mix diazepam and ketamine and give as bolus. In very depressed, recumbent animals or neonates, xylazine may be omitted. If sedation is considered necessary, 0.01–0.03 mg/kg butorphanol is recommended.
Xylazine/5% guaifenesin/ ketamine	0.5–1.1/"to effect"/ 0.75–2.2	Incorporating guaifenesin will help decrease xylazine and ketamine requirements.
Xylazine/5% guaifenesin/ thiopental	0.5–0.6/to effect/ 3.0–4.0	Thiopental can follow guaifenesin as a bolus or 2 g added to guaifenesin and given to recumbency.
Xylazine/Telazol	1.1/1.1	Reported to cause a more prolonged and slightly rougher recovery than xylazine/ketamine.

(continues)

Table 15–1   (Continued)

Agent/Protocol	Dosages (mg/kg)	Comments
Injectable anesthetic maintenance		Use following induction with xylazine-ketamine (with or without diazepam, butorphanol, or acepromazine).
Xylazine/ guaifenesin/ ketamine	0.5 mg/ml xylazine and 1 mg/ml ketamine added to 5% guaifenesin	"Triple drip": administered at approximately 2.2 ml/kg/hour May be used for induction of anesthesia (0.5–0.6 ml/kg) in horses weighing <200 kg.
Guaifenesin/ thiopental	2 mg/ml added to 5% guaifenesin	Can be used following induction with xylazine-ketamine or guaifenesin-thiopental. Anesthetic depth becomes more difficult to assess if the former is used. Avoid using more than 2 g thiopental for maintenance to minimize risk of rough recovery.

Foals

Induction/short-duration maintenance

Butorphanol/ diazepam	0.06/0.06 IV	Induce anesthesia by mask or nasotracheal intubation, preferably with isoflurane (or sevoflurane).
Butorphanol/ diazepam/ ketamine	0.06/0.1/2.2	Xylazine (0.2–0.5 mg/kg) may be added for healthy foals when they resist restraint or a painful procedure is to be performed. Duration of anesthesia: 10–20 min.
Analgesic options		Dosage intervals are guidelines to be tailored to individual patients based on ongoing assessment.
Buprenorphine	0.005 IM, SC	Interval: 6–12 hr
Butorphanol	0.02 IV, IM	Interval: 2–4 hr
Morphine	0.2 IM	Interval: 4–6 hr
		The presence of pain obtunds the excitatory response that can occur with morphine administration to horses; however, agitation and excitement can occur, which are controlled by xylazine (0.2–0.4 mg/kg IV).

(continues)

Table 15–1 *(Continued)*

Agent/Protocol	Dosages (mg/kg)	Comments
Morphine *(cont.)*	0.1 (epidural administration)	May be used alone or combined with xylazine or detomidine (see dosages in Table 3–4) for pain relief as far forward as thorax for 8–24 hr. Avoid formulations that contain the preservative formalin (the preservative methylparaben is acceptable). Use of the preservative-free preparation (Duromorph™) is optimal but, due to the low concentration, adequate dosage may be difficult to deliver due to the large quantity required.
Fentanyl (transdermal)	Two 100 μg patches per adult horse (applied over thorax behind elbow)	Duration of effect: 48 hr.
Phenylbutazone	2.2–4.4 IV, PO	Interval: 12 hr
Flunixin meglumine	1.1 IV	Interval: 8–12 hr
Ketoprofen	1.1–2.2 IV	Interval: 12–24 hr

Note: Dosages are most commonly administered IV.

*Draft breeds rarely require more than 600 mg (total IV dose) xylazine premedication for ketamine induction.

advisable but unnecessary to remove shoes prior to anesthetic induction; shoes with toe clips or devices that may cause significant body injury or excessive slipping during recovery should be removed. Covering shoes left in place with padding and tape will help minimize these risks.

Adequate preanesthetic sedation is essential in adult horses. Induction of anesthesia in an inadequately sedated animal will increase the risk of injury to both horse and handler. The most commonly used drug is xylazine. Combining a second agent with xylazine, such as butorphanol, acepromazine, or diazepam, will help assure a smooth induction (see Table 15–1). Avoid xylazine (at least high dosages) in foals less than 1 month of age if other agents are available (see Table 15–1). The induction agent most commonly used is ketamine, alone or in combination with guaifenesin or diazepam. Thiopental also is used, largely dependent on experience with the drugs and the occasional contraindication associated with ketamine in individual patients (e.g., head trauma, descemetocoele). As a general rule, protocols using ketamine produce a more reliable and smoother recovery; however, some animals—such as excitable, hot-blooded breeds, donkeys, mules, and ponies—may fail to respond to ketamine induction and short-term maintenance, making it necessary to use other or additional agents for induction and maintenance. Donkeys and mules appear sensitive to the effects of guaifenesin; incorporating guaifenesin into the induction protocol is effective, but care must be taken to avoid high-end dosages, which could precipitate apnea.

Because their response to anesthetics can be unpredictable, placing a catheter in the jugular vein, either before or after premedication, will provide easy access to administer additional drugs when needed to smooth induction, prolong the anesthetic period in field situations, and quickly obtund voluntary movement during inhalation anesthesia.

Intubation is performed blindly in the horse, with the head, neck, and back extended in a straight line. Inserting a speculum, such as a short piece of PVC pipe with the edges smoothed, will facilitate passage of the tube between the cheek teeth into the larynx. Once the tube reaches the larynx, it is retracted slightly, rotated 90°, and advanced again until it can pass by the arytenoid cartilages and "fall into" the trachea. This may need to be repeated, rotating in the same direction, one or several times before the tube bevel can pass into the trachea.

Endotracheal tubes also can be passed nasally; this practice is common in foals to facilitate an inhalant induction and may be indicated in adult horses for procedures of the oral cavity. Desensitizing the floor of the nasal opening with lidocaine jelly will facilitate tube introduction into the ventral nasal meatus. The disadvantage of nasotracheal intubation is that a smaller tube must be used, which will increase resistance to breathing. Orotracheal tube sizes range from 10 mm ID (newborn foals) to 30 mm ID for draft breeds. For nasotracheal intubation, 8–12 mm ID is used in foals and 16–20 mm ID can be passed in adult horses. Intubation is unnecessary during parenteral anesthesia. However, horses are obligate nasal breathers, and some individuals may develop stridorous inspiration during general anesthesia, which may require placement of an ET tube (nasal is convenient) to maintain airway patency. Appropriately sized tubes always should be available for quick intubation should a respiratory emergency develop.

Halothane, isoflurane, and, most recently, sevoflurane are used in horses. Halothane historically has been the agent of choice for elective procedures, due to its effectiveness and lower cost, despite a greater negative effect on cardiac performance and greater likelihood of hypotension. Isoflurane is a better choice for high-risk patients (e.g., those with colic or needing a cesarean section) and foals. Reports have suggested a rougher recovery associated with isoflurane anesthesia when used in relatively healthy horses. This potential undesirable effect can be minimized by administration of a sedative or tranquilizer (e.g., alpha$_2$ agonist, butorphanol, acepromazine) at the low-end dosage range, IV or IM, in the postoperative period. Intramuscular administration will provide a longer duration with less negative cardiovascular effects but should be given 15–30 min prior to the recovery period. Sevoflurane has been reported to produce smooth recoveries, even in healthy patients, due to its lower solubility (compared to isoflurane and halothane) and rapid clearance.

Supportive care considerations include adequate padding and proper positioning to minimize risk of myopathy and neuropathy, crystalloid fluid administration to counteract the hypotensive effects of inhalant anesthetics, provision of mechanical ventilation during inhalant anesthesia (especially for respiratory-compromised patients and during prolonged procedures), and administration of inotropic agents when indicated. Minimizing downtime is a critical factor in decreasing the risk of myopathy in all horses and especially important in large breeds, such as draft horses. The most commonly used inotrope in horses is dobutamine, administered "to effect" at an approximate infusion rate of 2–5 μg/kg/min. An easy method is to add 50 mg of dobutamine to a 500 ml bag of 0.9% saline or 5% dextrose and administer at a rate of 1–2 drop/sec (10 drop/ml drip set for adults; 60 drop/ml set for foals) until the desired blood pressure is achieved. Dobutamine may be used intermittently as needed or the administration rate can be adjusted to maintain a stable and adequate mean arterial pressure. Greater accuracy is provided by use of a syringe pump when available.

During parenteral anesthesia, the eyes should be covered to minimize external stimulation, the halter removed to minimize risk of damage to nerves lying superficially in the head, and oxygen supplemented (10–15 L/min) for procedures anticipated to exceed 60 min. Demand valves, which function at 50–80 psi to deliver 200–280 L/min of oxygen, provide supplemental and emergency ventilatory support for large animal patients during injectable anesthesia and recovery from inhalation anesthesia when an anesthesia machine is not readily accessible. The demand valve, connected to the endotracheal tube, is triggered by negative pressure created by the animal's spontaneous breath or manually by the operator. It adds resistance to breathing and should not be left on the ET tube for prolonged periods of time. It can be used connected to a stomach tube with the tip placed in the nasopharynx, but this is less efficient.

Vigilant monitoring is important in horses, as voluntary movement, sometimes without obvious warning, is common. Horses may exhibit transient apnea in the immediate postinduction period, which will delay anesthetic uptake if ventilatory support is not provided. Respiration is easy to observe in horses by direct visualization of the thorax and rebreathing bag. Normal rates should be 6–12 breaths/min, higher for foals (12–20 breaths/min). Horses are prone to hypoventilation and hypoxemia during anesthesia. Although of minimal consequence during short field procedures, these changes can become significant and affect cardiac performance during prolonged procedures. Arterial blood gas analysis, when available, will help guide ventilatory support and optimize homeostasis during the intraoperative period and is advised for procedures in excess of 60 min and for high-risk patients.

The heart rate (HR) tends to remain stable in adult horses (25–50 beats/min; performance animals may have even lower rates), even when anesthesia is inadequate, so it is not an effective indicator of anesthetic depth. Foals are the exception: a marked increase in HR is likely to occur during inadequate anesthesia. Invasive arterial blood pressure monitoring is a reliable and necessary monitoring tool during equine inhalation anesthesia to assure adequate perfusion pressure (minimal mean arterial pressure >60–70 mmHg, which will help minimize the risk of myopathy), provide information on cardiac performance, and signal inadequate anesthetic depth, with a sudden and rapid increase in pressure often (but not always) preceding voluntary movement. Both of the noninvasive arterial blood pressure monitoring techniques (Chapter 6) are applicable for short anesthetic duration (<1 hr) and seem to be especially effective in foals, although less reliable and accurate.

Eye signs used to assess inhalant anesthetic depth in horses include the palpebral reflex, which should remain slow but present; rapid nystagmus, which often signals impending movement (slow nystagmus may persist in some individuals without accompanying voluntary movement); and tearing, which may signal a light plane of anesthesia. These signs should be assessed in conjunction with cardiopulmonary parameters whenever critical assessment of anesthetic depth is made.

Recovery following inhalant anesthesia should occur in a dark and padded enclosure. Recovery may be assisted with a tail rope and halter if there is adequate room in the recovery area for personnel to escape injury and a method to secure the ropes. Assisted recovery is especially indicated for patients at risk of injury during recovery, such as orthopedic patients. Recovery is facilitated by placing animals on a large pad, to maintain padding, and to discourage attempts to stand until the animal is able. Postanesthetic sedation helps to delay attempts to stand until the animal can do so unattended or with minimal assistance. Two approaches to extubation are used, depending on personal preference and available facilities. The tube can be removed before swallowing is observed and replaced with a smaller nasotracheal tube, which should be taped *securely* to the muzzle to assure a patent airway throughout the recovery process. Or, the animal can be attended until swallowing is observed and then the tube removed, assuming a patent airway can be maintained at that time. Regardless of the preferred approach, oxygen supplementation (15 L/min) should be provided throughout recovery because a tendency to hypoxemia will persist until the horse returns to standing.

For field procedures, a safe and grassy area is preferred for recovery. The eyes should remain covered and the animal attended until it can be assisted to stand when a coordinated attempt is made.

16

Anesthetic Management of Ruminants and Camelids

Ruminants are amenable to standing chemical restraint and local techniques (Chapter 3) for a variety of procedures due to temperament (there are exceptions) and established effective restraint techniques. Table 16–1 lists dosages for agents to provide chemical restraint, induction, and parenteral maintenance of anesthesia. Anticholinergic administration is controversial and routine administration is not recommended. Bradycardia rarely is a complication of general anesthesia and administration of atropine will not significantly decrease salivation but will increase its viscosity and may contribute to development of bloat.

Table 16-1 Dosages of Injectable Anesthetic Agents Used for Chemical Restraint, Induction, and Maintenance of Anesthesia in Ruminants and Camelids

Agent/Protocol	Dosage (mg/kg)*	Comments
Ruminants		
Chemical restraint/ premedication		
Acepromazine		
Cattle	0.02–0.06	Ineffective alone for intractable patients.
Goats, sheep	0.04–0.08	May increase occurrence of regurgitation.
Diazepam (calves, small ruminants)	0.2–0.5	Minimally effective in adult cattle.
Xylazine**		
Cattle	0.01–0.1	In general, do not exceed 50 mg total dose; ↑ dosages may be required for intractable patients.
Goats	0.02–0.1	Do not exceed 0.02 (mg/kg) IM in kids.
Sheep	0.02–0.2	Hypoxemia due to pathologic pulmonary changes has been reported in sheep; if xylazine administration is unavoidable, use minimal recommended dosages and supplement oxygen while sedated.

Chloral hydrate		
Cattle	40–60 IV	Best used in combination with acepromazine or xylazine.
	80–100 PO, per rectum	
Goats	30–50 IV	
Butorphanol		
Cattle	0.01–0.04	
Sheep, goats	0.1–0.2	
Induction/ maintenance		
Thiopental (small ruminants)	10–15 IV	Induction of anesthesia.
5% Guaifenesin (cattle)	80–100 IV	When used alone for recumbency.
	50 IV	In combination with other agents.
5% Guaifenesin/ thiopental (cattle)	2–3 g added to 1 L 5% GG	Administered "to effect"; also may be used to maintain anesthesia short term. Add 3 g for cattle >1000 kg. Premedication usually unnecessary. Intubate animal during maintenance to avoid risk of regurgitation and aspiration.

(continues)

Table 16-1 (Continued)

Agent/Protocol	Dosage (mg/kg)*	Comments
5% Guaifenesin/ketamine (cattle)	2–3 g added to 1 L 5% GG	Add 3 g for cattle >1000 kg. Premedication usually unnecessary, but if needed for intractable patients, xylazine is effective. Induction dose: 0.5–1.0 ml/kg Maintenance dose: 2.2 ml/kg/hr ("to effect")
Xylazine/ketamine		
Cattle	0.04/2.2 IV	For ruminant neonates, use ≤0.02 mg/kg xylazine. Can mix and administer IV.
Goats	0.1 IM/5 IV	Xylazine should precede ketamine by 15 min.
Sheep	0.2 IM/5 IV	Xylazine should precede ketamine by 15 min.
Diazepam/ketamine	0.25/5 IV	Mix and administer IV "to effect." May require additional drugs especially if premedication is not administered.
Llamas		
Chemical restraint/premedication		
Xylazine	0.25–0.4 IV, IM	Lower dosage is for IV administration. Avoid in neonates; if necessary to perform minor procedures, use minimum dosage range and

Butorphanol	0.1–0.2 IV, IM	*only if* accurate weight is determined. Enhances sedation and analgesia with xylazine. Effective sedation for mask or nasotracheal induction or diazepam-ketamine induction in neonates and juveniles.
Induction/ maintenance		
Xylazine/ketamine	0.25/2.2 IV	Inject xylazine first then ketamine. For uncooperative animals, xylazine may be administered IM (0.4).
5% Guaifenesin/ ketamine	1 mg/ml ketamine in 1 L GG IV	1.1–1.6 ml/kg given "to effect" to facilitate intubation. This dose provides 15–20 min anesthesia and may be titrated to maintain anesthesia (if necessary).
5% Guaifenesin/ thiopental	2 mg/ml thiopental in 1 L GG IV	1.1–1.6 ml/kg given to effect to facilitate intubation. This dose provides 15–20 min anesthesia. Maintenance with this combination is not recommended.

(continues)

Table 16-1 (Continued)

Agent/Protocol	Dosage (mg/kg)*	Comments
Ruminants and camelids		
Analgesia		Dosage intervals are guidelines only: administration should be based on ongoing assessment.
Buprenorphine (small ruminants)	0.005 IM	Interval: 12 hr.
Butorphanol		
Cattle	0.01–0.02 IV, IM	Interval: 2–4 hr (or as indicated by patient).
Sheep, goats	0.1 IV, IM	
Morphine		
Sheep, goats	0.1 IM, SC	Dose should not exceed 10 mg. Interval: based on patient (every 6–8 hr?).
Ruminants, camelids	0.1 (epidural administration)	Provides analgesia as far forward as thorax for 8–24 hr. Due to the systemic side effects of epidural xylazine in ruminants, it is not recommended to add xylazine to morphine for long-term pain management, however if

indicated for additional analgesia, dosage for cattle and camelids is listed in Table 3–5.

Avoid formulations that contain the preservative formalin (the preservative methylparaben is acceptable). Use of the preservative-free preparation (Duromorph™) is optimal, but due to the low concentration and cost, adequate dosage may be difficult to deliver due to the large quantity required for adult cattle and camelids.

NSAIDs are not routinely used in ruminants; administration may be based empirically on equine dosages and used sparingly.

Phenylbutazone	
Cattle	2.2 IV, PO
Sheep, goats	5–10 PO
Flunixin	0.5–1.0 IV

*Drugs may be administered IM or IV unless otherwise indicated. Lower dosages should be utilized for IV administration.

**Great variation exists among breeds and individuals. Brahman breeds and Herefords may demonstrate increased sensitivity to xylazine effects and low-end dosages should be utilized and increased as needed.

Fasting is essential in ruminants and camelids (see Table 1–4) to decrease rumen/forestomach contents and thus decrease risk of regurgitation and aspiration, bloat, and respiratory compromise during induction and maintenance of general anesthesia. Neonates (less than 1 month of age) need only a 2–4 hr fast.

The need for premedication to facilitate catheter placement and anesthetic induction depends largely on patient cooperation and availability of restraint facilities (adult cattle). Agitated adult cattle will benefit from premedication regardless of secure restraint facilities to provide maximal safety to the animal and personnel and minimize movement during catheterization. In field situations, it may be necessary to cast the animal with ropes to facilitate handling following sedation. Small ruminants and calves can be adequately restrained by placing them in lateral recumbency, controlling the dependent limbs, and applying gentle pressure to the head and neck. Camelids have a unique personality and are prone to spitting, striking, biting, and butting. Placing a towel loosely over the face (hooding) will aid handling and help avoid being spit on. Adult camelids, like cattle, may be restrained in a chute or head gate. Premedication is indicated in all but the most tractable or debilitated camelid patients.

Vascular access in adult cattle and camelids is the jugular vein. Both species require cutdown via a stab incision through the skin to allow entry of the stylet and smooth passage of the catheter shaft. The jugular furrow is apparent and the vein usually easy to observe when occluded distally in cattle. However, in camelids, there is no discernible jugular groove and the vein does not become readily apparent, even when distally occluded, although a fluid wave may be observed with percussion. The optimal site for catheter entry into the internal jugular vein in camelids is the right side (to avoid the esophagus) at the junction of the cranial and middle third of the neck. There is greater risk of accidental penetration of the carotid artery compared to cattle. The jugular vein is used for small ruminants, calves, and young camelids and cutdown usually is unnecessary; additionally, the cephalic vein, similar in location to dogs, can be utilized.

Induction of anesthesia should be performed with rapid-acting agents (see Table 16–1) in adult ruminants and camelids to facilitate quick-sequence intubation and minimize risk of regurgitation and aspiration. Mask induction and maintenance with inhalant anesthesia is acceptable for ruminant and camelid neonates for short procedures (<1 hr). In adult cattle, intubation is performed by digitally palpating the arytenoid cartilages and guiding the ET tube through the larynx. When there is inadequate room for the hand *and* ET tube, passing a smaller long tube (a medium-sized equine nasogastric tube) digitally into the trachea, to guide passage of the ET tube, may be necessary. Rotation of the tube to manipulate the bevel will facilitate passage into the trachea. The cuff then should be inflated quickly to protect the airway.

Orotracheal intubation of small ruminants, camelids, and calves requires visualization of the larynx. A flat, long blade (180–350 mm) laryngoscope facilitates the procedure. Positioning of the endotracheal tube may obstruct the view of the ET tube passing through the larynx; passing a small, long, stiff piece of polyethylene tubing visually into the trachea to guide the ET tube may be beneficial in these cases. Use gauze loops to hold the mouth open and extend the head and neck to maximize visualization.

Blind orotracheal intubation is possible in llamas, small ruminants, and calves but more difficult than the procedure in horses. Nasotracheal intubation has been described for llamas and calves, and it also is more difficult than the procedure in horses. Llamas have a large pharyngeal diverticulum, which may complicate nasotracheal intubation. Head and neck extension is essential for both techniques. Delivering 1.0–2.0 ml of lidocaine through the tube with the tip positioned just over the larynx may help obtund swallowing and facilitate successful intubation.

Endotracheal tube sizes for adult cattle range from 20–30 mm ID and for adult camelids, 12–14 mm ID (10–12 mm ID for nasotracheal intubation). Calves and crias usually require size 8–12 mm ID and size 7–9 mm ID, respectively. Small ruminants accommodate size 8.0–12 mm ID tube, while juveniles require size 5.0–7.0 mm ID tube.

Adult ruminants and camelids should be positioned with support under the neck so that the head will tilt downward to prevent accumulation of saliva in the oropharynx and encourage drainage out of the oral cavity. Adequate padding of the down surface, positioning of the down forelimb forward and supporting the up limbs parallel to the table are necessary in adult cattle and camelids during prolonged procedures to minimize risk of myopathy and neuropathy. When adequate padding is not feasible, placing an inner tube tire around the down limb will help minimize risk of neuropathy. Small ruminants and neonates should be provided an external heat source for prolonged invasive procedures. Intraoperative fluids are indicated for prolonged procedures in all ruminants to replace intraoperative fluid losses and provide a route for administration of adjunct drugs.

Recovery in ruminants usually is uneventful; animals generally recover quietly and smoothly. Endotracheal tubes should be removed when swallowing is observed, with residual cuff inflation to remove any saliva or regurgitation that may have collected rostral to the cuff. Adult ruminants should be positioned upright in sternal recumbency as soon as possible, to facilitate eructation of collected rumen gases. Analgesic dosages are available for ruminants and should be administered when indicated (see Table 16–1).

17

Anesthetic Management of Swine

Swine anesthesia presents a plethora of challenges, including resistance to physical restraint, which often precludes adequate physical examination and collection of blood for preoperative assessment; lack of easily accessible superficial veins, which makes IV anesthetic induction challenging; difficult intubation; a tendency toward intraoperative hyperthermia, including an inability to dissipate heat due to low body surface to mass ratio and the risk of malignant hyperthermia; and lack of readily palpable peripheral pulses, which increases the challenge of effective intraoperative monitoring.

Pigs usually resist restraint. Neonates and companion breeds (i.e., Vietnamese potbelly) usually can be restrained by holding the animal against the body and wrapping with a towel. Safe restraint is critical in companion breeds to avoid damage to their relatively fragile skeleton. Restraint techniques used in food animal breeds, such as nose snares and lifting by the rear limbs, is not recommended. An effective device for restraining pigs of all sizes is a webbed stanchion with wheels to allow transport (Figure 17–1). Using a board or moveable gate to squeeze pigs into a small confinement usually facilitates IM premedication injection in larger swine.

Pigs vomit and an adequate fast (see Table 1–4) is important to minimize risk of regurgitation, especially when intubation is not planned. It is best to delay anesthesia, when possible, if fasting status is unknown or inadequate.

Intramuscular induction is the most common method of anesthesia in swine. The minimal needle length for injection is 11/2 in. to reach the muscle, since swine have a large quantity of superficial fat stores. Sites include the neck muscles just behind the ear and the muscles of the hind limb; the latter site should be avoided in pigs destined for human consumption. Intravenous induction by use of the auricular vein is possible following adequate premedication and restraint (Table 17–1). Pigs that can be safely restrained are amenable to mask induction with inhalation anesthetic agents. Pigs *usually* accept the mask and transition smoothly with minimal movement (3–5 min). The process is facilitated by premedication (see Table 17–1).

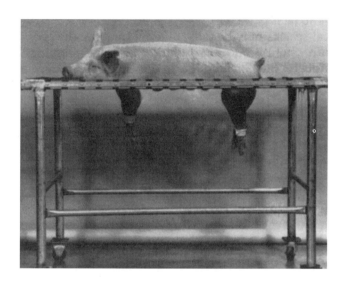

Figure 17-1 A web-topped mobile table for restraint and transport of swine for physical examination and induction of anesthesia. (Reprinted with permission from JC Thurmon and GJ Benson, Special anesthesia considerations of swine, in: *Principles and Practice of Veterinary Anesthesia*, CE Short, ed., Baltimore: Williams and Wilkins, 1987, page 311.)

Table 17-1 Anesthetic Agents for Premedication, Induction, and Analgesia in Swine

Agent/Protocol	Dosage (mg/kg)*	Comments
Chemical restraint/premedication		
Acepromazine	0.03–0.2	*Do not* exceed 15 mg. Minimal tranquilization.
Azaperone	0.4–3.0	Lower dosage range for larger swine; effects may persist for several hours.
Diazepam	0.4–1.0	Ineffective alone. Undependable absorption.
Midazolam	0.1–0.5	Quick onset. Minor effect when used alone.
Xylazine	0.5–2.0	Higher dosage for small swine and vice versa. Xylazine is less effective in swine than other species.
Medetomidine	0.01–0.05	Appears to be more effective than xylazine.
Butorphanol	0.1–0.2	May be combined with tranquilizer or alpha$_2$ agonist to enhance sedation.
Induction/maintenance		
Xylazine/ketamine	0.5–2.0/2.2–4.4	Induction is often prolonged and incomplete. Scale to pig size: Bigger pig takes lower dosage.

Xylazine/ketamine/ oxymorphone	2.0/2.0/0.075
	• Using medetomidine (0.02–0.04) in place of xylazine may provide a smoother, better quality induction.
	• Adding butorphanol may improve induction and quality of anesthesia.
	• In general, this protocol is inadequate for surgical maintenance; repeated dosing is necessary if movement persists.
	• Ketamine dose for PBP is 5–10 mg/kg.
	• For juveniles and PBP.
	• Good analgesia and muscle relaxation for minor surgical procedures; duration of effect is 20–30 min.
	• Rapid shallow breathing is a common side effect.
Xylazine/telazol	0.5–1.0/2–6
	• Provides rapid (<5 min) smooth induction.
	• Preferred induction agent but expensive.
	• Recovery may take several hours (>4 hr) when high-end dose is used.

(continues)

Table 17-1 (Continued)

Agent/Protocol	Dosage (mg/kg)*	Comments
		Medetomidine (0.02–0.04) may be used in place of xylazine, and butorphanol may be added to protocol.
		Provides adequate immobilization for minimally painful, noninvasive procedures.
Acepromazine/ketamine	0.1/5–10	Azaperone (0.4–2) may be substituted for acepromazine. Increase ketamine dosage to 15 mg/kg for PBP.
		Separate injections by 30 min, giving tranquilizer first.
		Unreliable; may provide adequate immobilization to gain IV access.
Thiopental	5–10 IV	Requires secure IV access, usually auricular vein.
		Use 2.5–5% solution to minimize tissue irritation at injection site.
		Excellent relaxation for intubation.
Guaifenesin (GG)/thiopental	Induction: 1.0 ml/kg IV	Add 2 g thiopental per 1 L of 5% GG.

	Maintenance: ≤4 ml/kg/hr IV	Delivery (ideally) should not exceed 1 hr to decrease risk of rough recovery.
Guaifenesin (GG)/ xylazine/ ketamine	Induction: 0.5–1.0 ml/kg IV	Add *1 mg/ml* xylazine *and 1 mg/ml* ketamine to 5% GG.
	Maintenance: 2.2 ml/kg/hr IV	Minimal respiratory depression.
		Recovery is smooth and relatively rapid even after 2 hr maintenance.
		Used for induction if IV access is possible or following IM induction (as previously outlined).
Telazol/ketamine/ xylazine listed	1.3–2.0 mg/kg (dissociative) (100 mg/ml dissociative)	Telazol (500 mg) is reconstituted with 2.5 ml each of ketamine and 10% xylazine. (The dosage equates to 1 ml/50–75 kg.)
		Also effective for PBP at a dose of 0.6–1.2 mg/kg dissociative, which equates to 0.006–0.012 ml/kg.

Antagonists

Alpha$_2$ receptor

Yohimbine	0.05–0.2 IV, IM
Tolazoline	1–2 IV

(continues)

Table 17–1 (Continued)

Agent/Protocol	Dosage (mg/kg)*	Comments
Atipamezole	0.2 IM	
Benzodiazepine		
Flumazenil	0.02–0.1 IV	
Opioid		
Naloxone	0.04 IV, IM, SC	
*Analgesia***		
Buprenorphine	0.005–0.02	Interval: 12 hr.
Butorphanol	0.1–0.4	Interval: 2–4 hr.
Morphine	0.2 IM	Interval: 4–6 hr.
	0.1 (epidural administration)	Interval: 12–24 hr.
		Morphine may be given alone (diluted to a volume of 3–5 ml with 0.9% saline) or added to lidocaine, with or without alpha$_2$ agonist, as described in Table 3–5.

Note: Dosages are also applicable for potbellied pigs (PBP) unless otherwise noted.

*Dosages are for IM injection unless otherwise indicated.

**Dosage intervals are extrapolated from other species. Administration ultimately should be based on ongoing patient assessment.

Pigs can be effectively maintained with inhalation agents delivered with a tight-fitting mask. However, for long and complicated procedures and in high-risk patients, endotracheal intubation is advised. Both sternal and dorsal recumbency have been recommended for swine intubation, with sternal being better when the experience of the anesthetist is limited. Intubation is difficult in swine for several anatomical reasons: The larynx is a long way from the tip of snout, the mouth does not open widely, there is a large middle ventricle (middle laryngeal ventricle) on the floor of the larynx and lateral openings near vocal folds (lateral laryngeal ventricles) that tend to trap the tip of the ET tube, and the larynx is susceptible to laryngospasm. To assist the process:

1. Use gauze strips (versus fingers) behind upper and lower canine teeth to hold the mouth open to optimize visualization.
2. Extend the head moderately.
3. Use a flat long-blade (180–350 mm) laryngoscope to visualize the larynx and pull the epiglottis forward.
4. Apply 2% lidocaine (0.2–0.5 ml) to the laryngeal opening to minimize risk of laryngospasm.

When the pig is positioned sternally, the tip of the tube should point ventral until it meets resistance as it contacts the floor of the larynx. The tube should be rotated 180° and advanced, with minimal pressure, just into the trachea, at which time the tube should be returned to the initial position and inserted to the appropriate level. Once proper placement is verified, the tube is secured with gauze, around the tube and then the snout, and the cuff inflated to form an effective seal. Tube sizes range from 3–4 mm ID in neonates up to 16–18 mm ID in large sows and boars, which is smaller (given comparable body weight) than for other species. Tube sizes for adult companion pigs usually are in the range of 5.0–7.0 mm ID.

For prolonged anesthetic procedures, an IV catheter should be inserted to provide fluid therapy and a route for administration of additional anesthetic agents when a parenteral protocol is being used. Sites include the auricular, cephalic (located on the dorsomedial aspect of the forelimb), femoral, and medial and lateral saphenous veins. Except for the auricular and femoral veins, these veins are difficult to visualize and successfully catheterize but provide alternatives when the auricular veins are too small to visualize (many potbelly pigs have small ears) or have hematomas due to unsuccessful catheterization attempts.

Effective monitoring devices include esophageal stethoscopes and capnometers (if intubated), ECG, and pulse oximeter on the tongue (if accessible), or ear (in nonpigmented individuals). Breathing rate should range from 8–20/min but may be higher in neonates. Heart rate should stay above 40–50 beats/min and usually is maintained at 70–100 when dissociative agents have been administered. Rates of 100–140 beats/min are common in neonates. Pulse quality can be assessed by palpation of femoral, brachial, metatarsal, coccygeal, and auricular arteries.

Temperature should be closely monitored in swine because of greater tendency to develop hyperthermia and increased susceptibility to malignant hyperthermia (MH). White breeds historically have been linked to the disease—specifically, Pietrain, Landrace, Hampshire, and (less commonly) Duroc. While hyperthemia following isoflurane anesthesia has been reported in a potbelly pig, the existence of genetically linked MH has not been demonstrated in this breed.

Malignant hyperthermia is an inherited predisposition to uncontrolled generalized muscle rigidity triggered by stress, *all* inhalant anesthetics (halothane has been the most commonly incriminated), and succinylcholine. The genetic defect is at the level of the sarcoplasmic reticulum and associated with excessive calcium release. Clinical signs include muscle rigidity, tachycardia, hyperthermia, tachypnea, metabolic acidosis, hypoxia, and blotchy skin. The disease can rapidly progress to dyspnea, apnea, arrhythmias, and death if not treated immediately. Treatment includes *discontinuation of inhalant delivery*, efforts to cool the animal (alcohol bath, chilled IV fluids), continued delivery of 100% oxygen to meet increased metabolic demands, bicarbonate administration (1 mEq/kg) preferably guided by blood pH analysis, corticosteroids, and dantrolene (2–5 mg/kg IV). Dantrolene is a peripheral muscle relaxant that suppresses calcium ion release from the sarcoplasmic reticulum but has minimal effect on respiratory muscle function. Oral dantrolene is less expensive than the IV preparation. Administration (5 mg/kg PO) 8–10 hr before anesthetic induction in high-risk breeds may be beneficial, especially when inhalant anesthetics must be used and a prolonged anesthetic period is anticipated.

Recovery in swine generally is uneventful and should take place at a neutral ambient temperature in a quiet, safe area. Small patients may require an external heat source, the need for which should be based on body temperature recorded at the end of anesthesia (see Table 6–3). Animals should be monitored until extubated and able to maintain sternal recumbency unassisted with normal vital signs.

18

Overview of
Cardiopulmonary Resuscitation

Prevention of cardiopulmonary arrest through appropriate patient preparation (minimizing risk factors) and optimal anesthetic management and monitoring is far better than cardiopulmonary resuscitation (CPR). Guidelines for CPR are summarized here. Resuscitation usually is successful in relatively healthy small animals (and large animal neonates) when arrest is recognized early; resuscitation in horses and adult cattle often is ineffective, making prevention through early recognition of and intervention for potential problems critical in these species.

Quickly recognizing signs of impending cardiopulmonary arrest is optimized by monitoring vital signs at

5-min intervals. Indications include cyanosis (which cannot occur in anemic patients if [Hgb] <5 g/dl); prolonged capillary refill time (CRT) (>2–3 sec); irregular, absent, or sudden change in pulse or heart sounds; cardiac arrhythmias; abnormal respiratory pattern or apnea; and loss of corneal reflex. When problems are noted, the first step is to stop delivery of anesthesia, flush the breathing system with 100% oxygen; and support ventilation to ensure adequate oxygen delivery. The ET tube should be checked for patency and the animal intubated if a tube is not already in place. When reversible agents have been used, administration of their antagonist is usually indicated.

CPR guidelines include basic (A, B, C) and advanced (D, E) steps for life support:

Step A. *Airway* Establish or assure patent airway with ET tube for delivery of ventilation.

Step B. *Breathing* Provide 100% oxygen (150 ml/kg/min for small animals; 15–20 ml/kg/min for large animals); ventilate *simultaneous with* chest compressions at a rate of 12–20/min (6–12 for large animals).

Step C. *Circulation (compressions)* Deliver chest compressions at 80–120/min (40–80/min or as rapidly as possible for large animals) in a "coughlike" manner, meaning rapid and forceful delivery of pressure. *Chest compressions should be initiated as soon as absence of effective blood flow is identified and*

while the airway is being assured or established.
External massage promotes forward movement
of blood through one of two methods. In small
patients or those with narrow thoracic width,
the *cardiac pump theory* best explains forward
blood flow associated with actual compression
of the myocardium during chest compressions.
In larger patients, the *thoracic pump theory*
explains the resulting forward blood flow as a
result of sudden and significant increases in
internal thoracic pressure (associated with
compressions) being transmitted to the heart.
Therefore, for small animals (<10 kg), compress the chest directly over the heart with
hands or fingers applied to both sides of the
chest. For larger patients (>10 kg), compress
chest over widest portion or at the seventh
intercostal space at the junction of dorsal and
middle thirds of chest. Ventral-dorsal compressions may be more effective in some patients.

In advanced CPR, step D includes *drugs and/or defibrillation* and step E is recognition of the specific *ECG*
abnormality. The initial drug to be administered is epinephrine followed by atropine and other agents (Table
18–1), as indicated by the individual patient's underlying
and identified problems and abnormalities identified on
ECG. Defibrillation is indicated for ventricular tachycardia and fibrillation and recommended dosages are listed
in Table 18–1.

Table 18–1   Dosages and Indications for Drugs Used During Cardiopulmonary Arrest

Agent Drug	Dosage(mg/kg)*	Indications/Effects
Epinephrine (IT)	0.02–0.2** (small animal) 0.01–0.02 (large animal)	Alpha agonist effects increase peripheral resistance and intrathoracic blood flow to promote perfusion while preferentially preserving flow to brain and heart. Beta activity to improve contractility and to reestablish normal cardiac rhythm (in some cases).
Atropine (IT)	0.02–0.04 (small animal) 2–6 mg total dose (large animals)	Increases heart rate. Treats bradycardia and asystole.
Lidocaine (IT)	2–4 (dogs) 0.5–1.0 (cats, horses, ruminants)	Treats recurrent ventricular arrhythmias and tachycardia.
Doxapram	0.05–0.2 (bolus) 5–10 μg/kg/min (infusion)	Central acting respiratory stimulant indicated for apnea due to anesthetic overdose.

Inotropes		
Dobutamine	2–10 µg/kg/min	Improves cardiac contractility once NSR is reestablished.
Dopamine	5–10 µg/kg/min	Direct renal vasodilatory effect (questionable in cats).
Ephedrine	0.03–0.1 IV bolus	Lower dose range for large animals. Increases heart rate in refractory cases.
Isoproterenol	0.01–0.1 µg/kg/min	Improves contractility but may decrease blood pressure due to beta₂ vasodilatory effects. Arrhythmogenic: monitor ECG during administration.
Calcium (chloride or gluconate)	5–10 mg/kg (small animal) 2 mg/kg (large animal)	Positive inotrope, may enhance effect of inotropic agents but can cause asystole if overdosed. Calcium has been incriminated in the pathogenesis of postresuscitation syndrome (cerebral ischemia) and is *not* used in resuscitation *(unless the underlying cause of arrest is due to hypocalcemia or hyperkalemia)*.

(continues)

Table 18–1   (Continued)

Agent	Dosage(mg/kg)*	Indications/Effects
Bicarbonate	1–2 mEq/kg or dose on calculated deficit†	Corrects metabolic acidosis. Usually unnecessary if arrest is <10 min and no underlying imbalance was present. Administration may promote more successful response to defibrillation. If administered when ventilation is inadequate, can promote intracellular acidosis (paradoxic cerebral acidosis) due to generation of carbon dioxide.
Corticosteroids		
Solu-medrol™ (methylprednisolone sodium succinate)	30	Protect against cerebral edema following resuscitation. Enhances ATP release from the mitochondria to facilitate normal membrane function.
Solu-delta-cortef™ (prednisolone sodium succinate)	30–60	

DexamethasoneSP (sodium phosphate)	2.0–4.0	
Electrical defibrillation	(watt-sec = Joule)	For ventricular tachycardia and fibrillaton.
External	5–10 Joule/kg	
Internal	0.5–2.0 Joule/kg	When electrical defibrillator is unavailable.
Chemical defibrillation		
Potassium chloride plus	1 mg/kg	Efficacy is questionable.
Acetylcholine	6 mg/kg	
10% Calcium chloride	10 mg/kg	Calcium follows KCl-acetylcholine mixture.
Postresuscitation therapy for cerebral protection		
Corticosteroids	As listed previously	
Furosemide	1 mg/kg	More effective in treating edema following mannitol.

(continues)

Table 18–1 (Continued)

Agent	Dosage(mg/kg)*	Indications/Effects
Mannitol	1 gm/kg	Cerebral edema; give over 20–30 min.
Diazepam	0.1–0.2 0.5 mg/kg/hr infusion	Given "to effect" to control seizures.
Propofol	1 mg/kg bolus 0.1 mg/kg/hr infusion	Seizure control; animal usually remains conscious at this dosage.

NSR = normal sinus rhythm.

*Drugs should be given intravenously *or* intratracheally (IT), *if* specified by the specific drug. Dosages for the IT route should be double the IV dosage. Dosages are in mg/kg unless otherwise specified.

**This dosage is controversial. Low dose suggests diluting epinephrine (1 mg/ml) with 9 ml of 0.9 saline and administering at 1 ml per 5 kg; high dose suggests use of undiluted epinephrine at 1 ml per 5 kg. It is prudent to attempt use of low dose epinephrine for one or two doses before utilizing the higher recommended dosage.

†Bicarbonate requirements are calculated by this equation:

Required amount (mEq/L) = Deficit (base deficit or difference between bicarbonate value and normal value) × BW (kg) × 0.3 (ECF volume). Give approximately one quarter the calculated deficit and reassess blood pH and gas values.

Intravenous access should be established early in the resuscitation efforts. While a central line (jugular vein) is ideal, a peripheral vein usually is easier and faster to access (at least in small animal species). Other routes for drug administration include intratracheal (epinephrine, atropine, lidocaine, naloxone) and intraosseous routes (also for fluid delivery). For intratracheal delivery,

1. Dose should be doubled.
2. Drug should be diluted in 3–10 ml of sterile saline or water.
3. Drug should be deposited with a small long catheter (urinary catheter) with the tip positioned at the carina.
4. Two or three breaths should be delivered immediately following drug instillation before resuming compressions.

Potential causes and specific treatment for electrocardiogram traces identified during arrest are listed in Table 18–2.

Internal cardiac compression has been shown to be more effective than external compression in promoting myocardial and peripheral tissue perfusion during CPR. Internal compression requires a thoracotomy, although cardiac access may be gained through the diaphragm when arrest occurs during an abdominal procedure. Indications include the presence of pneumothorax or

Table 18–2 Electrocardiogram Tracings Identified During Cardiopulmonary Arrest, Potential Predisposing Causes, and Treatment Steps

Trace	Potential Causes	Treatment Steps (in addition to steps A, B, and C)
Ventricular fibrillation	Excitement during induction or recovery (endogenous catecholamine release)	Early defibrillation (3 consecutive shocks)
	Anesthetic overdose	Reassess ECG, repeat counter-shock at increased level.
	Underlying myocardial disease or trauma	Administer epinephrine: low dose initially then high dose if no response; repeat shock.
	Undetected overpressurization of breathing circuit	Lidocaine for refractory cases; repeat shock.
	Hypothermia, hypovolemia	Identify and correct potential underlying causes.
	Acidosis or electrolyte imbalance	
Ventricular tachycardia	Same as for fibrillation	Treat like fibrillation if no palpable pulse.
		If pulse is palpable, lidocaine bolus.
Asystole	Anesthetic overdose	Low-dose epinephrine, atropine.

| | Hypotension: shock, endotoxemia Vagal stimulation: visceral, ocular | High-dose epinephrine. Administer fluid bolus (10–20 ml/kg). Dopamine if rhythm returns but pulse weak. Identify and correct underlying causes. |
| Electromechanical dissociation (pulseless electrical activity) | ECG may appear normal or show idioventricular or ventricular escape rhythm with *no* associated pulse Causes: hypovolemia, tamponade, pneumothorax, pulmonary embolism, hypoxia, anesthetic overdose | Same as for asystole. Administer corticosteroid early Consider bicarbonate after 10 min. Prognosis is poor for successful resuscitation |

broken ribs, inability to apply effective external compressions due to size and shape of the thorax, failure of external compression to produce effective forward blood flow, and absence of spontaneous rhythm after 5–10 min CPR. Thoracotomy is performed, following abbreviated aseptic preparation, by making a liberal incision at the fifth intercostal space. The pleura is penetrated with a finger or blunt tip to avoid damage to underlying thoracic structures. Compression rate should be coordinated with ventricular filling. Once spontaneous stable rhythm is reestablished, the thorax should be flushed with warm isotonic crystalloid fluid, the incision closed in a routine manner, and thoracocentesis performed to evacuate the pleural space.

Animals successfully resuscitated following CPA remain vulnerable to recurrence of myocardial instability and development of neurologic consequences associated with tissue ischemia and reperfusion insult. Oxygen supplementation should be continued and the ECG and arterial blood pressure monitored for several hours following resuscitation. Conservative fluid therapy (50 ml/kg/24 hr; less for cats) should be continued to maintain adequate perfusion and preload but minimize risk of contribution to edema formation. Glucose-containing fluids are *contraindicated* because glucose can exacerbate neurologic damage. Inotropic support may be necessary (see Table 18–1) and a suggested goal of therapy is to maintain diastolic blood pressure above 60 mmHg. Monitoring urine output provides an additional indicator of adequate tissue perfusion. Ideally, arterial pH and blood gas analysis should be performed to assure adequate ventilation and oxygenation and assess the metabolic acid-base status. When conscious, the animal's neurologic status should be evaluated and findings recorded. Cerebral edema may develop 24–48 hr following resuscitation and may be signaled by seizures, depression, coma, or blindness. Specific treatment for cerebral insult and edema are listed in Table 18–1.

Appendix 1

Approximate Dosages (mg/kg) of Anesthetic Agents and Adjuncts for Common Domestic Species

Drug	Dog	Cat	Horse	Cow	Sheep, Goat	Pig
Atropine	0.02–0.04	0.02–0.04	0.004–0.01	0.01–0.02	0.04–0.06	0.04
Glycopyrrolate	0.01	0.01	0.002	0.002	0.005–0.01	0.003
Acepromazine	0.05–0.2	0.05–0.2	0.02–0.06	0.01–0.1	0.04–0.08	0.03–0.2
Azaperone	–	–	–	–	–	0.4–3.0
Diazepam	0.2–0.4	0.2–0.4	0.02–0.1	0.02–0.1	0.1–0.2	0.4–1.0
Midazolam	0.1–0.4	0.1–0.4	–	–	–	0.1–0.5
Flumazenil	0.01–0.02	0.01–0.02	–	–	–	0.01–0.08
Xylazine	0.2–1.0	0.2–1.0	0.2–1.0	0.01–0.1	0.02–0.2	0.5–2.0
Detomidine	0.0005–0.02	–	0.01–0.04	0.01–0.02	–	–
Medetomidine	0.01–0.04	0.01–0.06	0.005–0.01	0.01–0.04	–	0.01–0.05
Romifidine	0.01–0.04	–	0.03–0.08	0.01–0.02	–	–
Yohimbine	0.05–0.15	0.1–0.2	0.07–0.1	0.2–1.0	0.1–0.2	0.05
Tolazoline	0.5–2.0	1.0–2.0	0.5–2.0	2.0–3.0	2.0–3.0	1.0–2.0
Atipamezole*	0.07–0.2	0.2–0.4	0.15–0.4	0.01–0.1	0.01–0.2	0.1–0.2
Morphine*	0.2–0.6	0.2–0.4	0.05–0.2	–	0.1–0.2 (10 mg max.)	0.2
Meperidine	2.0–6.0	5.0	2.0–4.0	2.0	2.0 (200 mg max.)	2.0
Hydromorphone	0.2–0.4	0.1–0.2	–	–	–	–

Oxymorphone	0.1–0.2	0.05–0.1	0.02	—	—	0.02
Fentanyl	0.002–0.006	—	—	—	—	—
Buprenorphine	0.005–0.04	0.005–0.01	0.005	—	0.005	0.005–0.01
Butorphanol	0.2–0.4	0.2–0.4	0.02–0.04	0.01–0.04	0.1–0.2	0.1–0.2
Nalbuphine	1.0–3.0	1.0–3.0	—	—	—	—
Pentazocine	2.0	2.0–3.0	0.3–0.5	—	—	2.0
Naloxone	0.001–0.04	0.001–0.04	0.01	—	0.005–0.02	0.01–0.05
Nalmefene	0.001	0.001	—	—	—	—
Chloral Hydrate	—	—	5–30**	40–60 IV 80–100 PO	30–50 IV	—
Methohexital†	3.0–8.0	3.0–8.0	5.0–6.0	3.0–6.0	2.0–4.0	3.0–10
Pentobarbital†	30	30	3.0–10.0	14.0	20.0–30.0	10–30
Ketamine	2.0–10.0	5–20	2.2 (IV only)	2.2 (IV only)	5.0–15.0	2.0–12.0
Telazol	2.0–8.0	2.0–8.0	1.1 (IV only)	2.0–4.0 (IV)	2.0–6.0 (IV)	2.0–6.0 IM
Thiopental†	10	10	4.0–6.0	4.0–8.0	4.0–10.0	4.0–8.0
Propofol (bolus)	2.0–6.0	2.0–4.0	2.0–4.0	—	—	—
(infusion mg/ kg/min)	0.4	0.4	0.05–0.1	—	—	—

(continues)

Drug	Dog	Cat	Horse	Cow	Sheep, Goat	Pig
Etomidate	0.5–2.0	0.5–2.0	–	–	–	0.5–2.0
Guaifenesin	–	–	40–80	60–100	60–100	40–80
Pancuronium	0.02–0.04	0.02	0.08–0.12	0.04–0.1	0.005	0.05–0.12
Vecuronium	0.012–0.2	0.024–0.04	0.05–0.1	–	0.005	0.1–0.2
Atracurium	0.12–0.4	0.06–0.25	0.07–0.1	0.15 (llama)	0.005/hr (infusion)	0.5
cis–Atracurium	0.05	0.05	–	–	–	–
Edrophonium‡	1.0	1.0	0.25–0.5	0.5	0.5	0.5
Neostigmine‡	0.04	0.04	0.02–0.04	0.02–0.04	0.2–0.04	0.02–0.04
Pyridostigmine‡	0.2	0.2	0.2	0.2	0.2	0.2

*Recommended for IM use only, although these agents have been used intravenously.

**Recommendations suggest using chloral hydrate in incremental low dosages to achieve desired effect, which ranges from mild to profound sedation-hypnosis.

†All barbiturates should be titrated to effect. Pentobarbital is *not* recommended for anesthetic induction and maintenance in clinical practice as recovery is prolonged and respiratory depression may be significant. When used, the calculated dose is given *"to effect,"* approximately one quarter to one half is given relatively rapidly and the rest titrated slowly to the desired level of anesthesia. The horse dosage listed for pentobarbital is for sedation or control of seizures. A dose of 15–30 mg/kg of pentobarbital injected intratesticularly has been recommended for castration of large boars.

‡Reversal of neuromuscular blockade with acetylcholinesterase inhibitors should be preceded by an anticholinergic agent regardless of species. Response to these agents is highly variable, depending on the degree of blockade present when agents are given; therefore, the dosage recommendations should be considered guidelines and effectiveness of reversal should be based on use of the train-of-four response (should be returned to normal) with a nerve twitch stimulator. See the first three references in "Recommended Reading" for details regarding interpretation of monitoring with the nerve twitch stimulator.

Appendix 2

Drug Scheduling Classification and Guidelines for Storing, Dispensing, and Administering Scheduled Agents

Schedule	Agent Signification	Description	Examples
I	C-I	No accepted medical use. Major potential for abuse.	Heroin, marihuana, methaqualone
II	C-II	Approved medical uses but high potential for abuse leading to addiction.	All pure opioid agonists (e.g., morphine), cocaine, pentobarbital, amphetamine

(continues)

Schedule	Agent Signification	Description	Examples
III	C-III	Approved medical uses. High potential for abuse but less than that for C-II.	Thiopental, telazol™, ketamine, anabolic steroids
IV	C-IV	Approved medical uses. Less potential for abuse than C-III but addiction is possible.	Diazepam, midazolam, oxazepam butorphanol, pentazocine, chloral hydrate, methohexital, phenobarbital
V	C-V	Approved medical uses. Least potential for abuse of the scheduled agents.	Buprenorphine

1. To administer, prescribe or dispense scheduled drugs, veterinarians must be registered (initial application: form DEA-224) with and approved by the Drug Enforcement Agency of the United States Department of Justice (Headquarters: 1-800-882-9539).

2. To purchase Schedule II drugs for clinical use, triplicate order form DEA-222 must be filled out and sent to the supplier. Upon receipt of Schedule II drugs, appropriate quantity should be verified by dating and completing the order form.

3. Schedule III-V drugs do not require the triplicate order form. However, records of transactions should be maintained for two years by use of supplier's invoices or logbook, including date of receipt and quantities ordered and received.

4. The DEA license is valid for only one office where controlled substances are administered or dispensed. If multiple offices are used to administer and dispense controlled substances, each must be registered independently.

5. A record of transaction must be maintained for all controlled substances administered or dispensed and should include patient name and identification, with drug and amount used to account for all controlled substances.

6. Controlled substances stored in a clinic must be kept in a securely locked, substantially constructed cabinet or safe. Ideally, stock should be kept to a minimum and maintained within a two- or three-lock system.

7. When controlled substances are dispensed, a record of each transaction is required.

8. For the prescription of controlled substances II-V, it is necessary to be registered with the DEA but it is not required to keep records of those transactions. Prescriptions must be signed and include the address and DEA registration number. The prescription order should be precise, legible, and alteration proof. Clearly indicate refill authorization directions. Schedule II prescriptions may not be refilled.

Appendix 3

Suggestions for Anesthetic Preparation and Management of High-Risk Patients

General statements may be applied to all species. (For specific protocols, see species-specific chapters.)

Trauma Patients

Preparation

Treat shock

- Fluid/blood component therapy
- Corticosteroids

Assess lead II ECG throughout the anesthetic period

Assess thoracic/abdominal imaging
Establish baseline blood pressure
Calculate lidocaine dosage

Management

Plan a rapid induction to gain control of airway
Induce with ECG if possible (small animal)
Monitor arterial blood pressure throughout the anesthetic period
Be ready to provide arrhythmia treatment and inotropic support
Manage pain appropriately

Cardiac Patients

Preparation

Identify potential problems

- Lead II ECG
- Thoracic radiographs
- Echocardiography

Plan for potential problems

- Arrhythmias
- Hypotension

Management

Determine fluid needs (conservative with risk of volume overload)

Premedicate to minimize anxiety

Oxygenate throughout anesthetic period (including pre- and postop)

Assist ventilation to maintain normal $PaCO_2$

Monitor cardiovascular parameters quantitatively if possible

Respiratory Patients

Preparation

Preoperative assessment

- Thoracic radiographs
- Arterial blood gas analysis

Thoracocentesis (when indicated)

Preoxygenation (essential)

Rapid (IV) premedication and induction

Management

Supervise entire premedication and induction process

Assist ventilation throughout the procedure

Assess continuous ECG if possible

Evaluate arterial blood gases intraoperatively, if available

Facilitate a smooth and gradual recovery

Provide oxygen supplementation throughout the recovery period

Neurologic Patients

Preparation

Record preoperative neurologic exam findings
Treat cerebral edema if necessary

- Solu-medrol/Solu-cortef: 20–30 mg/kg IV
- Furosemide: 1–2 mg/kg
- Mannitol: 1 g/kg over 20–30 min

Assure normal fluid balance to maintain normal MAP

Management

Provide smooth induction with minimal physical restraint
Use conservative but adequate fluid therapy (avoid glucose-containing fluids)
Provide IPPV to maintain $PaCO_2$ at 30–35 mmHg
Monitor ABP to assure adequate cerebral perfusion
Avoid acepromazine and ketamine; isoflurane is the best inhalant to use
Monitor mentation postoperatively and assess neurologic status frequently

Cesarean Section Patients

Preparation

Administer fluid bolus preoperatively (10–20 ml/kg)

Prepare surgery site prior to induction

Preoxygenate

Administer premedications

- To minimize anxiety
- Choose reversible agents

Prepare to provide resuscitation for newborns

- Oxygen delivery
- Oropharynx suction
- Warmth
- Reversal agents (e.g., naloxone)
- Dopram
- Administer agents into umbilical stalk or sublingually

Management

Two general approaches to anesthetic management:

1. Rapid induction/intubation with propofol or diazepam-ketamine following neuroleptanalgesic combination; maintain on isoflurane or sevoflurane

(halothane is acceptable but more cardiodepressing)

2. Neuroleptanalgesia (ruminants may not require premed) plus regional anesthesia: epidural, line block, paralumbar technique (Table 3–5)

Monitor and maintain adequate ABP
Efficiency is essential to minimize time to delivery

Hepatic Disease Patients

Preparation

Assess chemistry panel for accompanying abnormalities

- Hypoproteinemia
- Hypoglycemia
- Coagulopathy (coagulation panel, bleeding time)

Assure adequate fluid balance
Avoid agents that depend on hepatic metabolism

Management

Choose reversible premedications (e.g., opioid)
Benzodiazepine use is controversial and is best avoided in the presence of hepatoencephalopathy
Propofol or etomidate are good small animal induction agents; guaifenesin-ketamine is suitable for large animals

Isoflurane is most sparing of hepatic blood flow and is agent of choice

Consider glucose-containing fluids and colloids when indicated

Renal Disease Patients

Preparation

Correct azotemia prior to induction
Assure normal fluid balance
Assess for accompanying disorders

- Anemia
- Hypoproteinemia
- Acid-base and electrolyte imbalances

Be prepared to minimize anesthesia time

Management

Choose a cardiac-sparing protocol: opioid-benzodiazepine, ketamine, low-dose propofol, isoflurane maintenance

Administer fluids intraoperatively: (10 ml/kg/hr)

Monitor ABP and urine production (normal: 1–2 ml/kg/hr)

Consider dopamine infusion: 2–5 µg/kg/minute

Geriatric Patients

Preparation

Geriatric = the last 20–25% of natural lifespan

- <10 kg dogs >11 yr
- 10–25 kg dogs >10 yr
- 25–40 kg dogs >9 yr
- >40 kg dogs >7.5 yr
- cats >12 yr

Physiologic changes

- Decreased metabolic rate
- Decreased maximal cardiac output
- Decreased alveolar gas exchange
- Decreased organ reserve including liver and kidneys
- Increased fat
- Decreased anesthesia requirements

Complete physical exam, blood workup, other diagnostic tests as indicated by physical exam findings

Management

Select reversible premedication with minimal cardiac and respiratory effects: opioid + benzodiazepine

Preoxygenate

Induction: mask, propofol, thiopental, diazepam-ketamine

Isoflurane or sevoflurane for maintenance

Consider local/regional techniques to spare requirements

Monitor ECG and ABP

Administer fluids at conservative rate

Support ventilation during anesthesia

Provide adequate analgesia and oxygen postoperatively

Neonates

Preparation

Considerations

- Age: ≤12 wks
- Increased metabolic demands
- Cardiac output is rate dependent
- Response to hypotension is less well-developed
- PCV and TP slightly less than adults
- More susceptible to hypothermia

  increased surface area to body mass ratio

  less body fat

  poorly developed thermoregulatory center

- Increased susceptibility to dehydration
    greater body water content
    less ability to concentrate urine
- Hepatic function not fully developed
    limited ability to metabolize drugs
    limited glycogen stores

Management

Select reversible premedication with minimal cardiac effects: consider anticholinergic premedication when drugs known to decrease HR are used (e.g., opioids)

Premedication: opioid + benzodiazepine

Induction: mask induction, propofol, diazepam-ketamine

Maintenance: isoflurane or sevoflurane, nonrebreathing system

Administer glucose-containing fluids (2.5–5%)

Provide external heat sources

Postoperative period: maintain oxygen delivery as long as possible and provide warm environment

Recommended Reading

Altman RB, Clubb SL, Dorrestein GM, Quesenberry K, eds. *Avian Medicine and Surgery.* Philadelphia: WB Saunders Co.; 1997.

Fudge AM, ed. *Seminars in Avian and Exotic Pet Medicine: Anesthesia and Analgesia.* Vol 7. Philadelphia: W.B. Saunders Co.; 1998.

Johnson-Delaney CA, Harrison LR, eds. *Exotic Companion Medicine Handbook for Veterinarians.* Lake Worth, FL: Wingers Publishing; 1996.

Muir WW, Hubbell JAE, eds. *Equine Anesthesia Monitoring and Emergency Therapy.* St. Louis: Mosby Year-Book; 1991.

Muir WW, Hubbell JAE, eds. *Handbook of Veterinary Anesthesia.* 2nd ed. St. Louis: Mosby Year-Book; 1995.

Seymour C, Gleed R, eds. *Manual of Small Animal Anaesthesia and Analgesia.* United Kingdom: British Small Animal Veterinary Association; 1999.

Short CE, ed. *Principles and Practice of Veterinary Anesthesia.* Baltimore: Williams & Wilkins; 1987.

Thurmon JC, Tranquilli WJ, Benson GJ, eds. *Lumb and Jones Veterinary Anesthesia.* 3rd ed. Baltimore: Williams & Wilkins; 1996.

Tully TN, Shane SM, eds. *Ratite Management, Medicine, and Surgery.* Malabar, FL: Krieger Publishing Co.; 1996.

Index

Page references with "t" denote tables; "f" denote figures.